D0710506

Alcoholism and Its Treatment in Industry

ALCOHOLISM AND ITS TREATMENT IN INDUSTRY

CARL J. SCHRAMM, Editor

THE JOHNS HOPKINS UNIVERSITY PRESS
Baltimore and London

HF
5549.5
A4
A4

Copyright © 1977 by The Johns Hopkins University Press

All rights reserved. No part of this book may be
reproduced or transmitted in any form or by any means,
electronic or mechanical, including photocopying,
recording, xerography, or any information storage and
retrieval system, without permission in writing
from the publisher.

Manufactured in the United States of America

The Johns Hopkins University Press, Baltimore, Maryland 21218
The Johns Hopkins Press Ltd., London

Library of Congress Catalog Number 77-4783
ISBN 0-8018-1973-3

Library of Congress Cataloging in Publication data
will be found on the last printed page of this book.

CONTENTS

45646

TABLES AND FIGURES

PREFACE

Alcoholism has always been one of America's most serious public health problems. Only recently, however, has special attention been focused on the largest single subpopulation of alcoholics—persons whose alcohol abuse is associated with or occurs at their place of employment. Our new concern with this subpopulation can easily be seen in the number of alcoholism treatment programs being organized by industry and governmental agencies to help job-holding alcoholics. Further, the proliferation of clauses in labor contracts on the rights of alcoholic workers, the efforts of government to encourage employers to identify and refer problem-drinking workers for treatment, and the developments in employers' health insurance coverage for alcoholics or in union health and welfare funds all point to the flurry of activity going on in this field.

Much of the growing concern for alcoholic workers can be attributed to the passage of the Comprehensive Alcoholism Act of 1970. This law established the National Institute of Alcoholism and Alcohol Abuse, which has watched over the growing commitment of the federal government to the responsible treatment of alcoholism. In addition to stimulating treatment and research in all phases of alcoholism, the institute has been especially attentive to the establishment of new models of identifying and treating problem-drinking workers. As a result of the success of several pilot projects dealing with alcoholic workers, the secretary of Health, Education and Welfare, Elliot Richardson, in his second special report to the Congress on Alcoholism and Health in 1973 recommended that Congress act to encourage programs for early identification of problem drinkers and alcoholics in business and industry.

> The magnitude of the costs to the Nation's economy stemming from problem drinking and alcoholism is staggering. It is imperative to encourage the wider establishment, in government as well as in the private sector, of types of programs that, with the cooperation of labor and management, have successfully restored substantial majorities of affected personnel to health and normal function. The economic benefits of effective early identification and treatment programs demonstrably outweigh the costs, and the human benefits are beyond evaluation.

A second reason for the growth of industrial alcohol treatment programs has been the emerging realization on the part of businessmen, managers, union leaders, and industrial physicians of the staggering amount of productivity lost because of alcoholism. One recent estimate places the annual cost of alcoholism to the economy at $9.3 billion in lost productivity alone. The dimension of the economic costs to the firm have been pointed to repeatedly in such commercial forums as the *Harvard Business Review, Forbes,* the *Wall Street Journal,* and *Fortune.* Similarly, labor leaders have directed their attention to protecting alcoholic workers from job loss through active support of treatment programs and through increasingly protective collective bargaining language regarding the rights and responsibilities of the alcoholic worker. At present, the AFL-CIO has made a formal statement of policy on alcoholism and has formulated model contract language. Other units of the organized labor movement have aggressive policy statements in writing and in force throughout the nation. Provisions in United Auto Workers contracts, for example, ensure an alcoholic worker the right to a full medical treatment regimen before he may be considered for termination.

Despite this activity, there is little scientific knowledge available to guide policymakers and persons charged with setting up and administering industrial treatment programs. The proliferation of graduate level courses, management seminars, union training programs, and hundreds of "short courses" of one kind or another on industrial alcoholism and its treatment have taught us that there is no uniform series of authoritative articles to use in approaching the question. This book hopes to fill the gap. The papers assembled here have grown from the editor's experience in developing teaching materials for a course at The Johns Hopkins Medical Institutions. His role in directing the largest multi-employer, multi-union clinic for employed alcoholics in the country has brought him into close contact with all of the contributors to the book.

The first four chapters, comprising Part I of the book, present a number of the most important issues being debated and discussed in the area of industrial alcoholism. The first chapter is an overview of theory and research that has developed regarding the work-related aspects of alcoholism and problem drinking. As such, it provides a guide to the literature and a review of issues of concern to the field.

Economic analysis of the problem of alcohol abuse continues to develop both as a separate academic enterprise and, in a more prosaic vein, as a means for justifying treatment programs by those involved in program development. In Chapter 2, Berry and Boland estimate the work-related costs of alcohol abuse to both problem-drinking workers and the market sector to be on the order of $10 billion. Its importance lies both in the methodology it develops for estimating the economic impact of chronic health disabilities that are highly illusory and difficult to measure, and for its use of the epidemiologic data developed by Cahalan and Room in economic analysis.

Industrial treatment programs have most often been fashioned around the premise that a unitary approach to identification and referral in any given employment should be equally effective in delivering treatment to all workers. In Chapter 3, Trice and Beyer present findings from a study of the application of a formal alcoholism policy in 71 federal civil service installations by supervisors according to the skill level of employees. They conclude that different means for implementing alcoholism policies are necessary for employees in high-status occupations, and suggest some ways in which implementation could be improved for lower-skill-level workers.

One of the most important developments in the organization of alcoholism services in industry has been the recognition of the important role that organized labor can play in the success of efforts to identify, refer, and treat alcoholic workers. In Chapter 4 Leo Perlis describes the evolution of union interest in alcoholic workers and discusses some well-founded suspicions held by many union officials regarding alcoholism programs, a problem that must be dealt with in establishing joint union-management efforts. As the head of the AFL-CIO's community action programs, Perlis sets out the official policy of organized labor on the question of how best to approach the known alcoholic and describes a plan of labor-management cooperation in establishing the operating industrial treatment programs.

Part II is concerned with the process of establishing and operating programs in industry and with evaluating their effectiveness. Chapters 5 through 7 are written by the persons responsible for establishing three of the most widely known and respected treatment programs in the nation, each of which represents a different approach and a different "style" of identification and treatment. In Chapter 5, Otto Jones outlines one of the most innovative approaches to industrial treatment, the INSIGHT program at Kennecott Copper in Salt Lake City. INSIGHT handles a wide range of problems experienced by workers, including drug addiction, family problems, and financial difficulties in addition to alcoholism. Chapter 6, by William R. Cunnick, Jr., and Edgar P. Marchesini, outlines a more conventional treatment program but one which shows the adaptability of the counseling regimen to the problems of predominantly white-collar workers. The success of the program of Metropolitan Life in reaching higher-status workers is particularly significant in light of Trice and Beyer's findings concerning the difficulties of identifying such employees. The third program, described by Msgr. Joseph A. Dunne in Chapter 7, is that of the New York City Police Department. Especially interesting is Dunne's description of the difficulty of establishing a counseling unit within the context of a large organization whose employees are, ideally, "the conscience of the community." Dunne also evaluates the program, showing that the behavior of officers improved substantially following treatment.

Evaluation of industrial alcoholism programs is becoming increasingly important with growing government support and the concomitant need to demonstrate that outcomes justify the expenditure of public funds. Richard L. Williams and Joseph Tramontana's approach to evaluation in Chapter 8 is one of suggesting rigorous skepticism in analyzing the results of a treatment effort. They outline the many problems of bias and difficulties in measurement that can invalidate evaluation studies and present a model for assessing program effectiveness.

Part III examines the Baltimore Employee Health Program (EHP), an experiment in treating employed alcoholics through a shared clinical facility sponsored and utilized by a consortium of 12 companies and agencies and the 15 unions representing the labor forces of the participating employers. The three chapters in this section are studies arising from the EHP project which will be of interest to the student of alcoholism treatment in industry and of characteristics of employed alcoholics.

In Chapter 9, Carl J. Schramm provides a synopsis of the EHP experience as well as a critical look at the most difficult problems in establishing a new treatment effort. In Chapter 10 Janet Archer describes the EHP treatment population and compares the social stability, work behavior, and job satisfaction of employed alcoholics with those of a comparison group of non-problem-drinking workers. Finally, in Chapter 11, Paul Schollaert applies discriminant analytic techniques to the EHP population to explore the relationship between the individual's job context, with particular reference to sanctions against heavy drinking, and the probability that he will become a problem drinker.

This volume owes much to the stimulation of the Office of Research and Development of the United States Department of Labor's Employment and Training Administration, which provided funding for the Baltimore experiment. The special attention of Ron Jones of the department is gratefully acknowledged. The editor also wishes to express his warm appreciation to Barbara Winkler for her assistance during the three years of the EHP project and for her coordination of the many activities involved in preparing the manuscript for this book.

Carl J. Schramm
Baltimore, Maryland
June, 1977

PART I

ONE / Occupational Alcoholism: A Review of Issues and a Guide to the Literature

JANET ARCHER

In the mid-1970s, the problem of alcohol misuse by economically productive members of society has become well established, and the barrier that the skid-row image of alcoholics has presented to recognizing its full dimensions has been largely overcome. Although definitions of alcoholism vary among researchers and clinicians, there is virtually unanimous agreement that problems related to the misuse of alcohol are a source of concern to our society. It has been estimated that nine million American men and women are alcohol abusers or alcoholics, no more than 5 percent of whom are inhabitants of skid row. An estimated 5 percent of the U.S. work force are alcoholic individuals, and almost another 5 percent are serious alcohol abusers (National Institute on Alcohol Abuse and Alcoholism 1971).

Attempts to gauge the economic costs of alcoholism and alcohol abuse have resulted in a wide range of estimates. However, on the basis of an analysis of six areas of behavior identified as sources of significant economic costs related to alcohol misuse, the National Institute of Alcohol Abuse and Alcoholism (NIAAA 1974) estimated a total loss to society of $25.37 billion in 1971 alone. More significantly, about 40 percent, or $9.35 billion of the total, was the cost of lost production of goods and services by alcohol-abusing members of the nation's work force.

Given that the major costs of lost productivity are borne directly by the employer, it might not seem surprising that about 34 percent of the major industrial and business corporations in the United States have adopted some form of program to provide assistance to problem drinkers (NIAAA 1974).[1] As recently as 1959, however, there were no more than 50 companies with formal programs in

1. The literature reviewed here is restricted to the area of occupational alcoholism and does not cover the epidemiological data on "problem drinking." Except where indicated with quotation marks, the term *problem drinker* is used interchangeably with *alcoholic* in this chapter.

full operation (Presnall 1967). This significant growth in only 15 years reflects the efforts of private foundations, universities, and government agencies strongly committed to the diffusion of work-based alcoholism treatment programs. Out of their activities and interest had emerged the subfield of industrial, or occupational, alcoholism.

The literature on occupational alcoholism is twofold: (1) reports, investigations, and evaluations of occupational programs; and (2) research into the problem of alcohol misuse by employed persons. There are several articles that provide a general overview of how the problem of alcohol abuse by workers is being approached in industry (Trice 1959; "The problem drinker in industry" 1966; Presnall 1967; Norris 1968; Raleigh 1968; Heyman 1971; Sadler and Horst 1972; Von Wiegand 1972). Two articles on the history and nature of occupational programs including the period since the creation of NIAAA are Roman and Trice (1976) and NIAAA (1974). Specific programs are described in Habbe (1969), Cline (1975), and Williams and Moffat (1975). Some company programs which have been evaluated systematically are those of Consolidated Edison (Franco 1957, 1960; Pfeffer and Berger 1957), American Cyanamid (Clyne 1965), the New York Telephone Company (Kamner and Dupong 1969), and Illinois Bell Telephone Company (Asma et al. 1971; Hilker et al. 1972).

Compared with reports and studies on treatment *programs,* the literature on the characteristics of the people treated is quite sparse. The best single source on research on the job behaviors of problem drinkers is Trice and Roman (1972). Additional references on employed problem drinkers and on industrial treatment programs can be found in three bibliographies: Cameron et al. (1974), which covers the full range of literature, including popular magazine and newspaper accounts; NIAAA (1973), which emphasizes occupational programs; and NIAAA (1972*a*), which contains several abstracts of articles on treatment programs in industry. Finally, the *Journal of Studies on Alcohol* (formerly the *Quarterly Journal of Studies on Alcohol*) (vol. 1, 1941) regularly publishes articles on research in occupational alcoholism, and the *Labor-Management Newsletter* (vol. 1, 1972) is a continuing source of information on current developments in the field.

The present review of the literature on occupational alcoholism begins with a summary of the history and evolution of work-based treatment efforts from the initiation of the first programs in the 1940s to the present emphasis on the broad-brush or employee assistance concept. Several issues of concern to the field are then discussed, with emphasis on differing conceptions of the problem drinker and appropriate strategies for identification and referral to treatment.

The review concludes with a description of research on the problem-drinking worker, including his job behavior and possible reasons for his abuse of alcohol.

HISTORY AND EVOLUTION OF OCCUPATIONAL ALCOHOLISM PROGRAMS

Company programs to assist the alcoholic worker have existed since the 1940s. Largely through the efforts of the National Council on Alcoholism (NCA), a voluntary organization established in 1944, and the Yale Center of Alcohol Studies (now at Rutgers University), established in 1941, a few pioneering companies—including Du Pont, Allis Chalmers, and Consolidated Edison—sought to identify the alcoholic worker and refer him to treatment.

The major thrust of arguments to persuade companies to adopt programs was that alcoholism was a health problem that primarily afflicted individuals who were in their middle service years, and hence persons in whom the company had a large investment. The demonstrated success of Alcoholics Anonymous (AA) was used to convince employers that workers could, in fact, be restored to prior levels of productivity. In most early programs, supervisors were briefed on the symptoms of alcohol progression and instructed to confront any worker so identified about his drinking and send him to the medical department for diagnosis. Referral was most often to AA (Smithers Foundation 1959; Henderson and Bacon 1953; Trice 1959).

In 1960, unsatisfied by the slow growth in company programs, the NCA recruited a staff experienced in the techniques of management consultation to encourage more employers to initiate occupational alcoholism programs. The Smithers Foundation also became involved in the area of occupational alcoholism, and its support led to the creation of the Program on Alcoholism and Occupational Health in the New York State School of Industrial and Labor Relations at Cornell University. The promoters were aided in their efforts by the encouraging results being achieved by companies with active treatment programs. The number of new programs increased more than sixfold during the 1960s (Smithers Foundation 1969).

Components of Occupational Programs

Preferred strategies for identifying workers and referring them to treatment have evolved since the first programs began in the 1940s. The key features of successful programs have been identified and discussed at length elsewhere (Trice and

Roman 1972; Habbe 1969; NIAAA 1974; Lotterhos 1975; Roman and Trice 1976). These include a written policy which states the procedures for identifying, confronting, and referring employees who may have a drinking problem. The policy should specify that its provisions are to be applied evenly throughout the work force, without regard to occupational status or position; it should specify the distribution of authority and responsibility involved in policy implementation, as well as the rights and responsibilities of workers with respect to alcohol use and abuse; and it should be disseminated throughout the work force to inform both supervisory and rank-and-file employees of the provisions and operation of the program and to encourage self-referrals. Additionally, successful programs establish specific channels within the organization to discharge the policy. Although the first-line supervisor most often initiates the confrontation, a program coordinator should be appointed, both to relieve the supervisor of the onus of total responsibility for handling a problem drinker and to provide specialized expertise in counseling and/or referral to treatment. Finally, supervisory and management personnel should be trained as to their responsibilities in implementing the policy (Trice and Belasco 1968; Belasco and Trice 1969), and union officials should be involved at all stages of program implementation (Trice and Belasco 1966; Belasco et al. 1969; Smithers Foundation 1970). Because of the importance of the cooperation and consent of the labor union to the effectiveness of any program involving employee welfare, joint union-management programs are seen as ideal, although they have been relatively rare to date.[2]

Since the early programs, the supervisor's role has been restricted to that of documenting absenteeism and decreased work performance instead of attempting to distinguish the signs and symptoms of alcoholism. When confronting the employee with his declining work performance, the supervisor informs the worker that help will be made available if he cannot himself deal with the source of his problem. Whenever possible, no mention is made of the suspicion of alcoholism, based on the view that management's sole concern is with work performance, and not with the private behavior of the worker. If the confronted employee desires help, he is sent to the alcoholism counselor or coordinator, who confers with him and recommends an appropriate course of action. While referral to AA still predominates in many programs, a number of alternative treatment

2. In part, the difficulty in establishing joint union-management programs lies in the parties' differing philosophies regarding alcoholism among workers. Unions are skeptical of the cost-benefit considerations that appear to motivate management to initiate programs, preferring to view alcoholism treatment as an extension of workers' benefits. The issue of union-management cooperation in alcoholism programs is discussed in depth by Trice and Roman (1972) and Roman and Trice (1976). For a statement of labor's policy on the question of occupational alcoholism programs, see National Council on Alcoholism (1973), as well as Chapter 4 in this volume.

resources are being used, including in-house programs, family counseling services, and union welfare programs. Additionally, many companies have extended health insurance benefits to cover the costs of limited-stay inpatient or residential treatment plans.

Strict confidentiality is maintained in the confrontation and referral. The employee is assured that his job security and opportunities for promotion will not be jeopardized if he avails himself of the assistance offered, consistent with the idea that alcoholism is a disease and hence to be treated like any other health problem. If performance does not improve and the employee fails to take advantage of the help offered, he may be subject to discipline and/or discharge. To ensure that the rights and responsibilities of identified workers are maintained and that the policy of confidentiality is strictly enforced, an increasing number of labor-management agreements are including contract language on alcoholism (Schramm, 1977).

Factors in the Success of Work-Based Programs

Companies that have adopted alcoholism programs have reported success rates of between 50 and 70 percent, with an average success rate of 66 percent for industry nationwide (Von Wiegand 1972). By contrast, a review of 22 evaluative studies of alcoholism treatment in nonwork settings revealed success rates ranging from 4 to 75 percent, with the majority of programs (interquartile range) averaging from 18 to 35 percent (Mandell 1971).[3] Trice and Roman (1972) summarize the evidence more specifically. If success is measured by rehabilitation (rather than simply job retention), it would appear that company programs have success rates of about 50 percent, compared with 20 percent for state hospital programs and 10 percent for efforts directed at police-court inebriates.

Beyond the promise of high success rates, the concept of industrial alcoholism programs has been enthusiastically supported by increasing numbers of state agencies and private foundations interested in alcoholism rehabilitation and treatment. A major reason is that work-based programs are seen as providing a unique possibility for early intervention into the problem-drinking cycle. While conventional treatment programs must wait for the alcoholic to come to them (usually only after the problem has progressed to the last stages), it is reasoned that company programs can identify alcoholics at an early stage through observing deteriorations in work performance. Moreover, the work place offers a preexisting structure for identification and referral in the form of the supervisory process. This structure is also seen as providing a legitimate basis for interven-

3. The problem of evaluating claims of treatment success because of differences in outcome criteria is discussed by Schramm and DeFillippi (1975).

tion, because declining work performance and excessive absenteeism represent a breach of the worker-employer contract.

A key factor in the apparent success of company programs is that referred clients are employed, by definition, and usually have had many years of service with their employers. Indeed, a variety of prognostic studies involving alcoholic clients of noncompany treatment centers have identified current employment and job stability as predictors of treatment success (Kissen et al. 1968; Kurland 1968; Gerard and Saenger 1966). It has been argued that a socially stable alcoholic—e.g., one employed, married, having children, and owning a house—is an excellent candidate for treatment because of his stake in recovery to protect his social wealth. Hence the employed alcoholic who is referred for treatment via a company identification program not only has a social stake (his job) but is also confronted with the threat of losing it unless he takes corrective action (Findlay 1972).

It is thought that the major clinical value of constructive confrontation is its ability to precipitate a crisis which undermines a significant rationalization for denying alcohol abuse—i.e., steady employment. Lindeman's theory of crisis intervention (1956) would suggest that confrontation with impaired job performance by an authority at work constitutes a psychological and/or social crisis for the employee; motivation for treatment is higher during this period of crisis than during periods of noncrisis; and motivation for treatment is greater to combat not only the poor performance but also the broader problem of alcohol abuse which brought it about.

Constructive confrontation has been used successfully in both noncompany and industrial programs. Historically, the position of many alcoholism therapists has been to regard the voluntary seeking of treatment as an indicator of patient motivation and, hence, of treatment success (Sterne and Pittman 1965). But studies of chronic public inebriates (a group with relatively little social wealth at stake) have shown that coercive or nonvoluntary referral to treatment is not necessarily an obstacle to treatment participation and success (Davis and Ditman 1963; Mills and Hetrick 1963; Gallant 1971). In reviewing a wide range of company alcoholism programs, Trice and Roman (1972) found that the results of rehabilitation efforts using the confrontation strategy "appear to be better than those of efforts under other conditions." Comparing employed alcoholics who were referred under confrontation with voluntary referrals to the same treatment center, Smart (1974) found that although the highly motivated volunteers did better on an overall improvement scale, both groups improved equally in drinking, and the "coerced" group showed significant improvement on a variety of work behavior measurements.

Federal Support of Occupational Alcoholism Programs

Stimulated by the "alcoholism industry,"[4] and as an outgrowth of concern in the late 1960s over the problem of drug addiction, Congress passed Public Law 91-616 (the Hughes Act), which in 1970 created the National Institute of Alcoholism and Alcohol Abuse to guide national efforts in combating alcohol problems. Among the divisions within NIAAA designed to deal with alcohol problems of special populations is the Occupational Programs Branch, whose target population is employed problem drinkers. The Occupational Programs Branch provides funding for work-based treatment efforts primarily in two forms: grants to provide consultation at the local level to encourage and assist companies and state and local governments in launching treatment programs, and funding for demonstration projects to explore alternative models and methods of reaching and treating problem-drinking employees (NIAAA 1974).

One consequence of the emergence of the federal government as a sponsor of occupational alcoholism programs has been a further shift in the emphasis of the preferred program. Before the creation of NIAAA, occupational alcoholism policies and programs, with few exceptions, were designed to provide assistance solely to the problem-drinking employee. On the basis of its survey of existing programs and of knowledge in the field, however, the Occupational Programs Branch (NIAAA 1972*b*) endorsed the "broad-brush" approach as the ideal strategy for occupational alcoholism programs.

Also referred to as the troubled employee or employee assistance concept, the broad-brush approach advocates extending the identification, referral, and treatment capabilities of the conventional program to provide assistance to all employees with poor work performance, whether their problem is related to alcohol or not. Responsibility for the confrontation is shifted from the supervisor to the counseling department and/or alcoholism coordinator. The supervisor need only perform his traditional role, i.e., observing the job performance of his employees. He is instructed to refer any and all job performance problems to the counseling service, where, with the employee's confidentiality protected, the nature of the problem and the best course of action will be decided (Wrich 1974). Although the employee is free to reject the services offered to him, he is informed that his future employment depends on his job performance, thus preserving the "crisis-precipitation" element of the constructive confrontation strategy.

Because many problems other than those associated with alcohol can cause

4. Trice and Roman (1972) use the label "alcoholism industry" to characterize the collection of agencies and professionals who design and implement alcoholism prevention and treatment programs as well as those who try to obtain financial backing to support such efforts.

diminished work performance, it is estimated that only about half of the referrals made under a troubled employee program will be problem drinkers (NIAAA 1972*b*). NIAAA believes, however, that the troubled employee strategy will yield a much greater penetration of the alcoholic population[5] than earlier approaches, in part, by avoiding the stigma of programs associated exclusively with alcoholism. Moreover, the extent to which employees with other types of problems can be assisted by the program is seen as an added benefit of the broad-brush approach. But the greatest value of the broad-brush approach is held to be its potential for helping workers with alcohol problems before their drinking becomes so severe as to be resistant to rehabilitation efforts. It is argued that, in contrast with other programs that wait for signs of alcoholism to appear before taking action, observation of deteriorating work performance offers the promise for earlier identification and referral to treatment.

The extent to which the broad-brush approach is really as novel as its proponents claim has been disputed (Roman and Trice 1976), since identification via absenteeism and impaired work performance antedated federal involvement in occupational alcoholism programs. This issue will be discussed more fully in the following section. It can be noted here, however, that the extension of occupational programming concepts to all problem employees *is* a novel approach, and as the preferred strategy of the major promoter of occupational programs today—the federal government—the employee assistance idea is already becoming a prominent feature of work-based strategies to reach and rehabilitate problem drinkers.[6]

THEORETICAL ISSUES IN OCCUPATIONAL ALCOHOLISM PROGRAM CONCEPTS

The field of occupational alcoholism is beset by a number of unresolved issues and problems, including difficulties in evaluating program outcomes, prospects for long-term financial backing after expiration of governmental demonstration funds, the cooperation of labor unions in program policy implementation, and the question of penetration. In their review of alcoholism in industry, Roman and

5. The penetration rate is the number of problem drinkers referred to the program during a given time period divided by the total number of problem drinkers in the work force during a given time period. A method for calculating penetration rates and the problems involved are discussed in Chapter 8 of this book.

6. For a collection of papers emphasizing the employee assistance concept, see Williams and Moffat (1975).

Trice (1976) cover these practical problems at length, considering deficiencies in the present state of research as well.

This section will concentrate on issues of a more theoretical nature. The models of alcoholism that have had the greatest influence in the field of occupation alcoholism will be discussed, first in general, and second in relation to the evolution of conceptions of problem drinking workers and of strategies for identification, referral, and treatment.

The Disease Model

The disease model of alcoholism, which was pioneered by E. M. Jellinek (1946, 1960), among others, did much to reorient earlier attitudes toward alcoholism and alcoholics. The model was officially accepted by the treatment community in 1956 when the American Medical Association defined alcoholism as a disease (Plaut 1967). The idea of alcoholism as a disease rather than a moral weakness was widely accepted by "helping" agencies and personnel seeking to redefine the alcoholic as an individual not responsible for his behavior and thus worthy of rehabilitation and treatment.

Essentially, the disease concept, or medical model, sees alcoholism as a cumulative process in which the individual drinker gradually increases his consumption over the years, from occasional to habitual intoxication, and ultimately to a state of complete physiological and psychological dependence on alcohol. This progression of steps or stages to total dependency, or "addiction," is accompanied by a progression of stages of social deterioration, marked by familial and marital disruption, antisocial acts, work and money trouble, drinking with social inferiors, etc. The similarity between the disease model of alcoholism and the viewpoint of Alcoholics Anonymous is not coincidental. Indeed, pressure from AA was a factor in the AMA's decision to classify alcoholism as a true medical disease (Siegler et al. 1968).

For researchers and clinicians using the medical model, identification of alcoholics is largely a diagnostic problem. Both physiological (Criteria Committee 1972) and psychiatric (Catanzaro 1967; Pokorney et al. 1971) symptomatologies have been elaborated.

Epidemiological and Sociocultural Perspectives

The disease/medical model of alcoholism has been attacked by numerous investigators representing a range of concerns. Critics include researchers who fault the model for its lack of explanatory power (Keller 1962; Clark 1975; Robinson

1972), its insistence that abstinence is synonymous with rehabilitation and recovery (Pattison 1966; Pattison et al. 1968), its failure to take proper account of sociocultural factors (Bacon 1963), and its implications for social policy (Seeley 1962; Hirsh 1967). A representative spokesman for epidemiologically oriented researchers of drinking behavior is Cahalan (1970), who argues that the disease model posits an evolutionary and deterministic progression of symptoms and outcomes that does not bear up under investigations of actual drinkers. Indeed, the findings of several epidemiological studies would appear to cast doubt on the unidimensional view of alcoholism progression represented by the disease model (Wanberg 1969; Edwards 1973; Knupfer 1967). These criticisms have led many investigators to abandon the term *alcoholism,* and to use problems associated with alcohol abuse, or "problem drinking," as the criteria of interest, rather than disease-model indicators such as loss of control and sneaking drinks to infer stages in the progression toward addiction (Cahalan and Room 1974). Similarly, the use of role performance criteria, rather than abstinence, as indicators of treatment success (Trice et al. 1969) avoids some of the problems associated with the disease conception of recovery from alcohol problems.

Within the field of industrial alcoholism, the disease model also has its critics, notably Roman and Trice. Drawing on labeling theory which arose out of the sociological study of deviant behavior (Schur 1971),[7] Roman and Trice (1968) are concerned with the interplay between the behavior of an alcohol abuser and societal reactions to his deviance. They point out that the disease model is in partial conflict with the goal of identifying early or middle-stage problem drinkers to which most occupational programs are committed. Not only does the disease model define the situation as one which is largely outside of the individual's control, thereby providing an excuse for deviant behavior to continue, but it also runs the danger of inappropriate labeling and, thus, of the self-fulfilling prophecy: "For persons who are labeled alcoholic and who do not successfully affiliate with Alcoholics Anonymous, the future may be marked by continuation of deviance to the point of total impairment" (Trice and Roman 1972).

Labeling theory is a specific formulation of the more general sociocultural model of alcoholism which emphasizes the importance of social norms and values in defining what is appropriate drinking, what is deviant drinking, and how both will be sanctioned by society (Pittman 1967; Bacon 1962; Whitehead 1975). In essence, the sociocultural viewpoint is less concerned with the etiological forces that produce problem drinking (e.g., biological factors in a person's

7. It should be pointed out that labeling theory is a controversial area in the sociology of deviant behavior. It too has its critics (Gove 1975).

ability to tolerate alcohol or to control his consumption) than with the social responses to problem drinking, which either encourage or dissuade it (Trice and Roman 1972).

Changing Conceptions of the Problem Drinker and of Strategies for Identification, Referral, and Treatment

The controversy over diverging models, or conceptions, of alcohol problems discussed above is reflected in the evolution of preferred strategies for organizing occupational alcoholism programs. The reliance of early programs on the disease model has been alluded to. Promoters encouraged companies to view the problem drinker as a sick individual who could be rehabilitated with appropriate medical attention and the psychological and social support provided by membership in AA. In fact, the strategy of constructive confrontation as used in occupational programs to precipitate a crisis that might cause the worker to recognize his problem and seek to eliminate it parallels the AA notion of the necessity of "hitting bottom" before motivation to stop drinking occurs (Roman and Trice 1976). That programs were located primarily in medical departments is a further indication of the influence of the disease model in earlier occupational treatment efforts.[8]

By contrast, the approach now recommended by NIAAA's Occupational Programs Branch relies more heavily on the sociocultural model.[9] The philosophy underlying the employee assistance strategy is that the de-emphasis of the supervisor's role and the masking of efforts to identify problem drinkers under a more general "troubled employee" rubric will help circumvent the social stigma associated with labeling workers as alcoholics, and hence will decrease the reluctance both of supervisors to make referrals and of workers to accept the assistance offered and even to enter the program on a voluntary basis. Moreover, NIAAA sees occupational programs as having more properly a personnel than a medical function, consistent with its greater emphasis on psychological and social factors in problem drinking. Although alcohol abuse is still treated largely as a health problem, with services frequently reimbursed through the worker's medical insurance plan, there appears to be a tendency away from referring to

8. For an illustration of the application of physiological criteria in the diagnosis of alcoholic employees, see Kamner and Dupong (1969) and Chapter 6 of this book. An example of a study of the psychiatric characteristics of employed alcoholics is Hurwitz and Lelos (1968).

9. There is evidence that the sociocultural model is gaining wide acceptance by occupation programming educators. For example, the lead article (Lotterhos 1975) in a recent collection of papers advocating the employee assistance concept makes explicit reference to labeling theory and its advantages over the disease concept in understanding problem drinking among workers.

alcohol problems in illness terms. For example, Wrich (1974) seems to prefer the terms "chemical dependence" and "chemical disorder" rather than "addiction," "alcoholism," or "disease."

Given that the medical model has been a useful device in encouraging employers to initiate programs, and given the demonstrated successes of the constructive confrontation strategy, one might wonder why the value of the medical approach is increasingly being disparaged by promoters of occupational programming concepts. Indeed, while it may be of limited applicability to behavioral science research, the therapeutic potential of the disease approach has had much greater exposure and, hence, more opportunity to be evaluated in the context of actual treatment than have the behavioral concepts underlying the sociocultural model.

In considering the role of these competing conceptions of alcoholism in the area of occupational programming, it is necessary to distinguish between members of helping agencies and services, whose primary motivation is to treat and rehabilitate problem drinkers, and researchers and scientists, whose ultimate goal is to enlarge scientific and/or clinical understanding of problem drinking. Although these groups overlap to a certain extent—as in the case of social scientists brought in by treatment foundations and agencies to serve as consultants, or in the case of company physicians using their treatment experiences to contribute to the research literature—their interests and motivations diverge. While scientists are likely to prefer testing their theories and confirming previous findings in a variety of empirical settings before recommending broad-scale applications, the helping agencies will tend to embrace or reject those very theories on the basis of their promise for achieving the "helping ends."[10]

In fact, given the optimism with which NIAAA viewed the potentialities of work-based programs when it first entered the field, it has been suggested that NIAAA's disapproval of earlier concepts is more apparent than real. Referring to NIAAA's endorsement of the broad-brush approach, Roman and Trice (1976) argue that

> advocates of the employee assistance strategy have attempted to strengthen the case for both the logic and the novelty of their approach by subtly posing earlier programs as being both narrow and naive. . . .
>
> The need for the employee assistance approach was justified on the basis that earlier

10. One example of this is the skepticism with which Roman and Trice view the employee assistance concept, even though part of the justification for that approach was based on inferences drawn from research studies which they and their colleagues conducted. Reviewing the problems and objections that have been raised in response to the troubled employee strategy, Roman and Trice (1976) conclude that its endorsement and promotion by NIAAA may have been premature.

programs . . . had been relatively unsuccessful. In point of fact, evaluative data from these earlier programs showed that they did indeed enjoy considerable success. . . , and there is no published evidence of program failures. This raises the question as to other possible motivations that may have led to the advocacy of the employee assistance strategy.

Roman and Trice go on to suggest some interesting possibilities. They argue that the employee assistance concept, by requiring a wide dimension of occupational program activities, would allow NIAAA to socialize the new "change agents" as professional consultants, who would meet with greater receptivity in work organizations than would the traditional alcoholism specialist with his "social worker" or "do-gooder" image. Moreover, by defining the employee assistance program as a personnel department function, the change agents could bypass altogether company physicians, who would be expected to reject encroachment by what they might perceive as lesser professionals.

Such a scenario might explain the peaceful coexistence of the notion of alcoholism as a health problem and the concomitant deemphasis on terminology traditionally associated with alcoholism treatment. This "latent function" of the employee assistant strategy is not entirely novel to NIAAA, however. As was discussed in the previous section, ten years earlier the National Council on Alcoholism had also sought to recruit a staff experienced in the techniques of management consultation to promote the growth of occupational alcoholism programs. It might be argued, then, that given the real-world priorities of program diffusion and implementation, the conceptions of the problem drinker and of strategies for identification and referral must accommodate empirical realities as well as, or perhaps in spite of, empirical research. Nevertheless, the modifiability of underlying philosophies can be easily overstated. For a different impression of the flexibility of preferred theories, models, and treatment concepts, one need only recall the outrage of the "alcoholism industry" in June 1976 ("Booze for alcoholics?" 1976) when the Rand Corporation made public its analysis of 45 NIAAA treatment centers nationwide, suggesting that some alcoholics can return to normal drinking.

RESEARCH ON ALCOHOLIC WORKERS

Despite the proliferation of the company treatment concept and its implementation nationwide, basic research into the job-related components of alcohol misuse and the work behaviors of problem drinkers occupies only a small space within the growing literature on industrial alcoholism. Indeed, an article in the U.S. Department of Labor's magazine, *Manpower* (U.S. Department of Labor 1970), concluded that the current state of knowledge and research on the problem did not provide an adequate basis for establishing public policy regarding drinking and the labor force.

This section discusses the research on job behaviors of alcoholic workers, causal factors in work roles, and the identification of alcoholics in company treatment programs.

The Impact of Problem Drinking on Job Behavior

Early investigations of the job behaviors of problem-drinking workers focused on absenteeism (Stevenson 1942; O'Brien 1949; Franco 1954), accidents (Trice 1957*a*), and bases for identifying problem drinkers on the job (Straus 1952; Trice 1957*b*). Comparing the absence and accident patterns of problem drinkers with those of normal employees, Observer and Maxwell (1959) found that alcoholics were absent 2.5 times more often and were three times more costly to their employers in sickness payments. In a study undertaken to aid in the early identification of problem-drinking workers, Maxwell (1960) investigated the kind of drinking symptoms which first appear on the job. Responses of recovering male alcoholics to questionnaires concerning their work behavior during the total problem-drinking period yielded a list of 44 on-the-job drinking symptoms. The predominance of diminished attendance and performance among the first signs of on-the-job problems to appear (8 of the first 20 signs) lent indirect support to more current emphases on early detection of problem drinkers through signs of impaired performance and absenteeism rather than through signs of alcoholism per se.

Another area of interest was the occupational stability of alcoholic workers. Throughout the 1950s there appeared a number of surveys of the social and occupational characteristics of alcoholic treatment populations showing the great majority of alcoholics to be socially and economically integrated members of society (Straus and Bacon 1951; Falkey and Schneyer 1957; Wellman et al. 1957; Chodorkoff et al. 1961). During the same period, reports on the experiences of operating company alcoholism programs were appearing in management and industrial medicine journals.[11]

Reviewing the evidence available from these surveys and studies, Harrison

11. For a review of this literature through 1958, see Trice (1959).

Trice (1962) summarized the basic data on the behavior of alcoholics that could be substantiated:

—The alcoholic works regularly while his malady is in its incipient and middle stages.
—Problem drinkers are rather evenly distributed through all occupational groups as well as many types of businesses and industries.
—The middle-stage alcoholic appears to be lodged heavily among male employees in the ages from 35 to 50 years.
—Work efficiency declines as alcoholism develops.
—In general, the absenteeism rate for a company's problem drinkers is significantly higher than for nonalcoholics.

From the continuing work of Trice and his co-investigators, and from other researchers as well, we now have a broader understanding of the work-related aspects of problem drinking, not only with respect to the impact of excessive drinking on specific job behaviors, but also with regard to how features of the work environment influence the expression of problem drinking.

In a study of the effects of problem drinking on job performance, Trice (1962) analyzed the work histories of 752 AA members through their own reports of their work behavior during the middle stages of their alcoholism. Trice also collected data from the AA members on three job variables—occupation, job freedom, and off-the-job drinking with co-workers—in order to examine the effects of features of the work experience itself. The data showed that almost all respondents experienced a substantial decrease in work effectiveness, and 70 percent indicated a progression of absenteeism during their problem-drinking period.

But Trice's study went beyond the confirmation of previous findings by showing that the amount of absenteeism and the nature of both impaired performance and absenteeism varies according to the occupational status of the employee. Professional, managerial, and other white-collar personnel tended to go to work even when they were intoxicated or hungover, but did practically nothing once there. Lower-status workers, on the other hand, tended to resort both to absenteeism and to further drinking off the job when in the same condition, but performed a substantial day's work whenever they were on the job.

Trice explained these findings as reflecting both a higher commitment to the job as well as a greater opportunity to cover up deviant drinking by higher-status employees. Indeed, higher-status workers, often having a greater degree of job freedom, reported that they themselves were able to cover up their drinking behavior. Workers in other occupational groupings, however, were more likely to rely on fellow workers or supervisors to cover up their drinking, or else to attempt no cover up at all. Findings on off-the-job drinking experiences with fellow workers showed high-status employees covering themselves there as well, being careful to drink normally while with work associates. By contrast, lower-status employees drank with a relative lack of inhibition when with co-workers.

Additionally, Trice found that job turnover among AA workers was not substantially higher than that of the labor force in general, thus confirming earlier findings that alcoholics work regularly in the early and middle stages of their affliction. Similarly, on-the-job accidents resulting in loss of time from work did not prove to be substantially greater than the norm among respondents, regardless of occupational type. Interview data revealed that when these workers were in poor physical condition, they took special precautions to prevent accidents, frequently resorted to absenteeism whenever they were more afraid of accidents than usual, were often removed from potentially dangerous jobs by supervisors, and were sometimes able to steady themselves by moderate on-the-job drinking.

For the most part, subsequent studies on the impact of problem drinking on job performance have expanded upon and/or confirmed earlier findings. Since Observer and Maxwell's study on sickness payments (1959), there have been a few studies and estimates of the economic loss to employers caused by problem-drinking workers (Winslow et al. 1966; Comptroller General 1970), as well as some insight into what an alcoholic on a bender might himself lose in wages and other expenses beyond the direct cost of alcoholic beverages (Babbitt 1967).[12]

Much of the confirmation of prior research came in a series of studies that Trice (1964, 1965*a*, 1965*b*) conducted to compare the job behavior of alcoholic, psychotic, neurotic, and normal employees and supervisors' reactions to their work. For example, when asked to respond to Maxwell's list of 44 signs of developing alcoholism, supervisors ranked lower work quality and lower work quantity as the fifth and twelfth most significant symptoms. Moreover, supervisors consistently gave alcoholics the lowest ratings of the three groups of problem employees. Trice also found that alcoholics did not have significantly more on-the-job accidents than the other employees, supporting both his earlier results on the accident experience of AA members as well as Maxwell's ranking of accidents as the most infrequent of 44 early signs of on-the-job drinking.

Findings from other populations of employed problem drinkers have also shown little evidence of frequent job turnover (Smart 1974; Warkov et al. 1965). Finally, Trice's findings showing variations in alcohol-related work behavior

12. The literature on the costs of alcohol abuse to the employer is reviewed by Trice and Roman (1972, pp. 2–9).

according to occupational position have also been confirmed—by Stamps (1965) as regards both cover-up and absenteeism and by Trice (1965*a*), Warkov et al. (1965), and Maxwell and Wasson (1963) as regards absenteeism.[13]

Causal Factors in Work Roles

Roman and Trice have paid the most explicit attention to etiological factors in work roles that may promote alcohol abuse. Their continuing investigations and reviews of populations of working problem drinkers has led them to postulate nine occupational risk factors in the job environment that appear to be conducive to the development and perpetuation of deviant drinking or drug abuse (Roman and Trice 1970). The nine factors, summarized below, are inherent in many high-status positions and tend to serve as barriers to the detection of deviant drinking. Roman (1974) argues that such jobs provide a setting for "successful deviant drinking" among middle- and upper-middle-level employees.

Lack of visibility:

1. jobs in which production goals are nebulous;
2. flexible work schedules and output permitting the exercise of an individual worker's option;
3. jobs which are remote from the purview of supervisors and work associates.

Stress factors stemming from the absence of structured work:

4. work addiction;
5. work role removal and occupational obsolescence;
6. job roles novel to the organization.

Absence of social controls:

7. job roles which require drinking as part of work role performance;
8. job roles in which one's deviant drinking benefits others in the organization;
9. mobility from a highly-controlled job status in which heavy drinking is practiced to release tension into a job status which is also stressful but in which social controls are absent.

With respect to features of the work environment that may be precursors or concomitants of problem drinking by persons in lower-status jobs, the evidence

13. Although Pell and D'Alonzo (1970) concluded that occupation appeared to have little influence on the excess absenteeism of alcoholics, their tabular data show the absenteeism frequency rates among unskilled workers to be considerably higher than those of workers in other occupational categories. Additionally, in a population not restricted to blue-collar workers (Maxwell 1972), stay-away absenteeism was the least frequent of four signs of alcohol-related deterioration in a group of 406 male recovered or "recovering" alcoholics.

is largely conjectural and comes primarily from researchers working, not in the area of occupational alcoholism, but in such fields as industrial sociology and mental health. For example, in a study commissioned in 1971 by the secretary of Health, Education, and Welfare to examine health, education, and welfare problems from the perspective of work, O'Toole et al. (1973) stated in summary: "A growing body of research indicates that, as work problems increase, there may be a consequent . . . increase in drug and alcohol addiction." The task force concluded that although no causal links have been established, the available evidence suggests the therapeutic value of meaningful work and improved working conditions for employees suffering from alcoholism and from other mental health problems. Similarly, McLean (1970) states that "workers with personality disorders, including alcoholism and drug abuse, may find that their psychiatric disorder stems partially from job insecurity, unpleasant working conditions or hazardous work." That a relationship may exist between alcohol misuse and unsatisfactory work experiences is suggested by a number of investigators in the sociology of work who have studied the effects of job dissatisfaction on general mental health. In his study of 407 automobile workers, for example, Kornhauser (1965) found that approximately 40 percent had some symptoms of mental health problems and that the major factor associated with positive mental health was job satisfaction.

Ironically, the general thrust of such arguments is that the source of much of the job discomfiture that may contribute to alcohol and drug dependency among lower-status workers lies in the absence of the very work-role features which Roman and Trice have found to be possible precursors of alcohol abuse by persons in high-status jobs. However, Roman and Trice have offered some suggestions as to how the highly structured, menial, and repetitive tasks of many blue-collar workers might contribute to alcohol abuse. They argue that the association found by McClelland et al. (1972) between heavy alcohol use and unmet power needs may be extended "to posit alcohol use as a coping device among those who have failed according to organizational or occupational criteria and who sense a gap between achieved and aspired power and status; McClelland's data likewise may apply to the attraction to alcohol among those who are forced to remain in low status jobs throughout their work career, always subject to the power of others in the organization" (Roman and Trice 1976).

While several suggestions have been made regarding a possible relationship between work-role stress factors and alcohol abuse, there is little empirical evidence available either to support or disavow them. Hardy and Cull (1971) compared the vocational satisfaction of 93 alcoholics and 72 nonalcoholics, using the occupations the former actually held before admission to a rehabilitation and treatment center. They found that alcoholics' job preferences were at variance both with the type of jobs they actually held, as well as with their abilities, while there was greater concordance between jobs held and job preference among the nonalcoholics. In another study of the possible effect of alcoholism on thwarting work ambitions, Hochwald (1951) reported that only 4 of 30 white alcoholic males interviewed had attained occupational goals they set for themselves in earlier life. Finally, in his study of 80 outpatients of an alcoholism clinic, Strayer (1957) measured occupational adjustment as a function of (1) ability to accept supervision, (2) relations with co-workers, and (3) work at the level of one's expressed occupational goal. In this instance, only 19 percent of the sample were functioning in accordance with their vocational goals.

Although the above studies would appear to suggest a relationship between alcoholism and the failure to achieve occupational goals, the fact that they did not take into account the occupational status or position of the workers limits the usefulness of their findings. Occupation has been found to be a more consistent predictor of how an individual will feel about his job than any other single variable (Robinson 1969). Moreover, only one of the studies had a comparison group of nonalcoholics, yet that group was not really comparable, having a greater proportion of white-collar workers than the alcoholic population.

In a study of blue-collar alcoholics in Baltimore, Schramm et al. (1976) found no significant differences between the alcoholics and a comparison group of normal males employed in the same work force, on a range of job satisfaction questions. However, there was evidence of a greater aspiration-achievement discrepancy among the alcoholics concerning broader life goals.[14]

The Identification of Alcoholics in Company Treatment Programs

With few exceptions, the study populations providing data on the job aspects of problem drinking are composed of workers who have been identified through company alcoholism programs. Large-scale samples of problem-drinking workers, such as Trice's population of AA members, are difficult and costly to secure, while company-identified problem drinkers constitute readily available, albeit imperfect, research populations. Moreover, since the government and private agencies providing most of the funding for work-centered alcoholism studies have been primarily interested in treatment results, those investigators concerned with developing basic data on the labor force behavior of problem drinkers have had to work with samples of workers that, while not necessarily representative of

14. These findings are described more fully in Chapter 10 of this book.

the problem-drinking labor force as a whole, are often the only ones available for study and evaluation.

Given the nature of the populations available for analysis, it is not surprising that much of the emphasis in the research literature on industrial alcoholism has centered on the mechanisms of company alcoholism identification, referral, and treatment systems.

The most notable feature of such systems has been their tendency to produce treatment populations composed primarily of low-status, blue-collar workers. For example, in Trice's comparative study of problem employees (1965*a*), alcoholics—in contrast to psychotics and neurotics—"were found in lower status job situations: less pay, fewer promotions, more dependents, less education, blue-collar jobs of a manual nature, requiring mobility rather than a fixed position." Warkov et al. (1965) conducted a study in a private utility firm with the primary purpose of investigating factors in the identification of problem-drinking employees. Comparing the characteristics of workers whom supervisors identified as having work problems due to drinking with those of a random sample of workers in the same firm, they also found that "[the] incidence of identification as a problem drinker varied inversely with social, occupational and organizational status of employees." This selection bias also results in differential rates of identification by occupational status in noncompany alcoholism programs. For example, with reference to employed alcoholics referred by Detroit courts to a state hospital for vocational rehabilitation, Ethridge and Ralston (1967) noted a "tremendous overrepresentation in the categories of service workers and laborers."

Since findings from large-scale samples indicate that neither alcoholism (Straus and Bacon 1951), "problem drinking" (Cahalan and Room 1974), nor heavy drinking (Cahalan et al. 1969) is restricted to any one social or occupational status grouping, it seems likely that the predominance of problem-drinking workers in lower-status occupations in company alcoholism treatment populations is an imperfect reflection of the epidemiology of alcoholism.[15]

Alcoholism scholars have observed that social class acts as a selecting factor, both for the identification of alcoholics and for the type of therapies they receive once in treatment (Schmidt et al. 1970). It has been found that middle-class alcoholics often go undetected by treatment personnel, while lower class alcoholics are readily identified as such (Blane et al. 1963). Trice's findings on

15. Epidemiological studies have, in fact, shown problem drinking to be more prevalent in the lower social classes. This differential, however, probably accounts for only part of the exceptionally high proportion of low-status workers in alcoholism treatment populations. This issue is discussed in detail in Chapter 3 of the present book.

problem-drinking job behaviors suggest an additional factor that may reinforce this tendency toward differential identification, i.e., the nature of the work role itself. Since white-collar, middle-class jobs are subject to less supervision, are less interdependent with the work of others, and afford more opportunities for "self-cover-up," the problem drinking of such higher-status workers is more likely to go unnoticed than that of blue-collar employees.

The tendency of supervisors in company alcoholism programs to identify and refer workers in predominantly low-status occupations has become a major concern among funders and promoters of such programs, since the uneven distribution of referred workers suggests that many problem drinkers are escaping identification and thus are going untreated. But given the paucity of systematic evidence obtained from truly representative populations, it is unrealistic to expect that workable solutions to such problems as the hard-to-identify alcoholic can be evolved at the present time. Nevertheless, research into the very phenomenon of differential selection for treatment has provided a number of suggestions for the development of theory on the relationship between problem drinking and features of the work environment which not only act as barriers to identification, but which may also hold the promise for a more thorough understanding of the problem of alcohol misuse in the work force.

REFERENCES

Asma, F., R. L. Eggert, and R. R. J. Hilker. 1971. "Long-term experience with rehabilitation of alcoholic employees." *Journal of Occupational Medicine* 13:581–85.

Babbitt, E. H. 1967. "What does it cost to be an alcoholic?" In D. J. Pittman, ed., *Alcoholism,* pp. 45–52. New York: Harper and Row.

Bacon, S. D. 1962. "Alcohol and complex society." In D. J. Pittman and C. R. Snyder, eds., *Society, Culture and Drinking Patterns,* pp. 78–100. New York: Wiley.

———. 1973. "The process of addiction to alcohol: Social aspects." *Quarterly Journal of Studies on Alcohol* 34:1–27.

Belasco, J. A., and H. M. Trice. 1969. *The Assessment of Change in Training and Therapy.* New York: McGraw-Hill.

Belasco, J. A., H. M. Trice, and G. Ritzer. 1969. "Role of unions in industrial alcoholism programs." *Addictions* 16:13–30.

Blane, H. T., W.F. Overton, and M. E. Chafetz. 1963. "Social factors in the diagnosis of alcoholism. I: Characteristics of the patient." *Quarterly Journal of Studies on Alcohol* 24:640–63.

"Booze for alcoholics?" 1976. *Time.* June 21.

Cahalan, D. 1970. *Problem Drinkers: A National Survey.* San Francisco: Jossey-Bass.

Cahalan, D., I. H. Cisin, and H. M. Crossley. 1969. *American Drinking Practices: A*

National Study of Drinking Behavior and Attitudes. New Brunswick, N. J.: Rutgers Center of Alcohol Studies.

Cahalan, D., and R. Room. 1974. *Problem Drinking among American Men*. New Brunswick, N.J.: Rutgers Center of Alcohol Studies.

Cameron, C., with D. Montgomery and S. Reilly. 1974. *Alcoholism and Work: Bibliography*. Madison, Wis.: Current Trends Retrieval.

Catanzaro, R. J. 1967. "Psychiatric aspects of alcoholism." In D. J. Pittman, ed., *Alcoholism*, pp. 31–52. New York: Harper and Row.

Chodorkoff, B., H. Krystal, J. Nunn, and R. Wittenberg. 1961. "Employment characteristics of hospitalized alcoholics." *Quarterly Journal of Studies on Alcohol* 22: 106–10.

Clark, W. B. 1975. "Conceptions of alcoholism: Consequences for research." *Addictive Diseases* 4:395–430.

Cline, S. 1975. *Alcohol and Drugs at Work*. Washington, D.C.: Drug Abuse Council.

Clyne, R. M. 1965. "Detection and rehabilitation of the problem drinker in industry." *Journal of Occupational Medicine* 7:265–68.

Comptroller General of the United States. 1970. *Substantial Cost Savings from Establishment of Alcoholism Programs for Federal Civilian Employees*. Report to the Special Subcommittee on Alcoholism and Narcotics of the Committee on Labor and Public Welfare, U.S. Senate. Washington, D.C.: U.S. Government Printing Office.

Criteria Committee, National Council of Alcoholism. 1972. "Criteria for the diagnosis of alcoholism." *American Journal of Psychiatry* 129:127–35.

Davis, M., and K. Ditman. 1963. "The effect of court referral and disulfram on motivation of alcoholics." *Quarterly Journal of Studies on Alcohol* 24:276–79.

Edwards, D. W. 1975. "The evaluation of troubled-employee and occupational alcoholism programs." In R. L. Williams and G. H. Moffat, eds. *Occupational Alcoholism Programs*, pp. 40–135. Springfield, Ill.: Charles C Thomas.

Edwards, G. 1973. "Epidemiology applied to alcoholism: A review and an examination of purposes." *Quarterly Journal of Studies on Alcohol* 34:28–56.

Ethridge, D. A., and J. A. Ralston. 1967. "Occupational backgrounds of institutionalized alcoholics: Comparative data and implications for rehabilitation." *Mental Hygiene* 51:543–48.

Falkey, D. B., and S. Schneyer. 1957. "Characteristics of male alcoholics admitted to a medical ward of a general hospital." *Quarterly Journal of Studies on Alcohol* 18:67–97.

Findley, D. 1972. "Anxiety and the alcoholics." *Social Work* 17:29–33.

Franco, S. C. 1954. "Problem drinking and industry: Policy and procedures." *Quarterly Journal of Studies on Alcohol* 15:443–59.

———. 1957. "Problem drinking in industry: Review of a company program." *Industrial Medicine and Surgery* 26:221–28.

———. 1960. "A company program for problem drinking: Ten years' follow-up." *Journal of Occupational Medicine* 2:157–62.

Gallant, O. 1971. "Evaluation of compulsory treatment of the alcoholic municipal court offender." In N. Mello and J. Mendelsch, eds., *Recent Advances in Studies on Alcoholism*, pp. 730–44. Washington, D.C.: U.S. Government Printing Office.

Gerard, D., and G. Saenger. 1966. *Outpatient Treatment of Alcoholism: A Study of Outcome and Its Determinants*. Toronto: University of Toronto Press.

Gove, W. R., ed. 1975. *The Labelling of Deviance*. New York. Halsted Press.

Habbe, S. 1969. *Company Controls for Drinking Problems*. Studies in Personnel Policy, no. 218. New York: National Industrial Conference Board.

Hardy, R. E., and J. G. Cull. 1971. "Vocational satisfaction among alcoholics." *Quarterly Journal of Studies on Alcohol* 32:180–82.

Henderson, R. M., and S. D. Bacon. 1953. "Problem drinking: The Yale plan for business and industry." *Quarterly Journal of Studies on Alcohol* 14:247–62.

Heyman, M. M. 1971. "Employer-sponsored programs for problem drinkers." *Social Casework* 52:547–52.

Hilker, R. R. J., F. E. Asma, and R. L. Eggert. 1972. "A company-sponsored alcoholic rehabilitation program." *Journal of Occupational Medicine* 14:769–72.

Hirsh, J. 1967. "The disease concept of alcoholism: Wish or fulfillment?" In J. Hirsh, ed., *Opportunities and Limitations in the Treatment of Alcoholics,* pp. 3–20. Springfield, Ill.: Charles C Thomas.

Hochwald, H. 1951. "The occupational performance of thirty alcoholic men." *Quarterly Journal of Studies on Alcohol* 12:612–20.

Hurwitz, J. I., and D. Lelos. 1968. "A multilevel interpersonal profile of employed alcoholics." *Quarterly Journal of Studies on Alcohol* 29:64–76.

Jellinek, E. M. 1946. "Phases in the drinking history of alcoholics: Analysis of a survey conducted by the official organ of Alcoholics Anonymous." *Quarterly Journal of Studies on Alcohol* 7:1–88.

———. 1960. *The Disease Concept of Alcoholism*. New Haven: Hillhouse Press.

Journal of Studies on Alcoholism. Rutgers Center for Studies on Alcoholism (previously Yale Center for Studies on Alcoholism).

Kamner, M. E., and W. G. Dupong. 1969. "Alcohol problems: Study by industrial medical department." *New York State Journal of Medicine* 69:3105–10.

Keller, M. 1962. "The definition of alcoholism and the estimation of its prevalence." In D. J. Pittman and C. R. Snyder, eds., *Society, Culture and Drinking Patterns,* pp. 310–29. New York: Wiley.

Kissin, B., S. Rosenblatt, and S. Machover. 1968. "Prognostic factors in alcoholism." *Psychiatric Research Reports of the American Psychiatric Association* 24:22–43.

Knupfer, G. 1967. "The epidemiology of problem drinking." *American Journal of Public Health* 57:973–86.

Kornhauser, A. W. 1965. *Mental Health of the Industrial Worker: A Detroit Study*. New York: Wiley.

Kurland, A. 1968. "Maryland alcoholics: Follow-up study I." *Psychiatric Research Reports of the American Psychiatric Association* 24:71–82.

Labor-Management Alcoholism Newsletter. National Council on Alcoholism, Labor-Management Division.

Lindemann, E. 1956. "The meaning of crisis in individual and family living." *Teachers College Record* 57:310.

Lotterhos, J. F. 1975. "Historical and sociological perspectives of alcohol-related problems." In R. L. Williams and G. H. Moffat, eds., *Occupational Alcoholism Programs,* pp. 3–39. Springfield, Ill.: Charles C Thomas.

McClelland, D. C., W. N. Davis, R. Kalin, and E. Wanner. 1972. *The Drinking Man.* New York: The Free Press.
McLean, A. 1970. *Mental Health and Work Organizations.* Chicago: Rand McNally.
Mandell, W. 1971. "Does the type of treatment make a difference?" Paper presented to the American Medical Society on Alcoholism.
Maxwell, M. A. 1960. "Early identification of problem drinkers in industry." *Quarterly Journal of Studies on Alcohol* 21:655–78.
———. 1972. "Alcoholic employees: Behavior changes and occupational alcoholism programs." *Alcoholism* [Zagreb, Yugoslavia] 8:174–80.
Maxwell, M. A., and J. Wasson. 1963. "Social variables and early detection of alcoholism on the job." Unpublished manuscript.
Mills, R., and E. Hetrick. 1963. "Treating the unmotivated alcoholic: A coordinated program in a municipal court." *Crime and Delinquency* 9:46–59.
National Council on Alcoholism. 1973. *Labor-Management Alcoholism Newsletter,* vol. 2, Jan.–Feb. Special labor edition.
National Institute on Alcohol Abuse and Alcoholism (NIAAA). 1971. *First Special Report to the U.S. Congress on Alcohol and Health.* U.S. DHEW Publication no. (HSM) 72-9099. Washington, D.C.: U.S. Government Printing Office.
———. 1972*a*. *Alcoholism and Rehabilitation: Selected Abstracts.* U.S. DHEW Publication no. (HSM) 72-9136. Washington, D.C.: U.S. Government Printing Office.
———. 1972*b*. *Occupational Alcoholism: Some Problems and Some Solutions.* U.S. DHEW Publication no. (HSM) 73-9060. Washington, D.C.: U.S. Government Printing Office.
———. 1973. *Subject Area Bibliography on Occupational Alcoholism Programs.* Rockville, Md.: National Clearinghouse for Alcohol Information.
———. 1974. *Second Special Report to the U.S. Congress on Alcohol and Health.* Washington, D.C.: U.S. Government Printing Office.
Norris, J. L. 1968. "Alcoholism in industry." *Archives of Environmental Health* 17:436–45.
O'Brien, C. C. 1949. "Alcoholism among disciplinary cases in industry." *Quarterly Journal of Studies on Alcohol* 10:268–78.
Observer and M. A. Maxwell, 1959. "A study of absenteeism, accidents and sickness payments in problem drinkers in one industry." *Quarterly Journal of Studies on Alcohol* 20:302–12.
O'Toole, J., chairman. 1973. *Work in America.* Report of a Special Task Force to the Secretary of Health, Education, and Welfare. Cambridge, Mass.: The MIT Press.
Pattison, E. M. 1966. "A critique of alcoholism treatment concepts, with special reference to abstinence," *Quarterly Journal of Studies on Alcohol* 27:49–71.
Pattison, E. M., E. B. Headley, G. C. Gleser, and L. A. Cottschalk. 1968. "Abstinence and normal drinking: an assessment of changes in drinking patterns in alcoholics after treatment." *Quarterly Journal of Studies on Alcohol* 29:610–33.
Pell, S., and C. A. D'Alonzo. 1970. "Sickness absenteeism of alcoholics." *Journal of Occupational Medicine* 12:198–210.
Pfeffer, A. Z., and S. Berger. 1957. "A follow-up study of treated alcoholics." *Quarterly Journal of Studies on Alcohol* 18:624–48.
Pittman, D. J. 1967. "International overview: Social and cultural factors in drinking

patterns, pathological and nonpathological." In D. J. Pittman, ed., *Alcoholism,* pp. 3–20. New York: Harper and Row.

Plaut, T. F. A. 1967. *Alcohol Problems: A Report to the Nation by the Cooperative Commission on the Study of Alcoholism.* London: Oxford University Press.

Pokorny, A. D., B. A. Miller, T. E. Kanas, and J. Valles. 1971. "Dimensions of alcoholism." *Quarterly Journal of Studies on Alcohol* 32:699–705.

Presnall, L. F. 1967. "Folklore and facts about employees with alcoholism." *Journal of Occupational Medicine* 9:187–92.

"The problem drinker in industry." 1966. In *Aspects of Alcoholism,* 2:45–50. Philadelphia: J. B. Lippincott.

Raleigh, R. L. 1968. "Alcoholism and industry." In R. J. Catanzaro, ed., *Alcoholism: The Total Treatment Approach,* pp. 393–400. Springfield, Ill.: Charles C Thomas.

Robinson, D. 1972. "The alcohologist's addiction: Some implications of having lost control over the disease concept of alcoholism." *Quarterly Journal of Studies on Alcohol* 33:1028–42.

Robinson, J. P. 1969. "Occupational norms and differences in job satisfaction: A summary of survey research evidence." In J. P. Robinson, R. Athanasiou, and K. B. Head, eds., *Measures of Occupational Attitudes and Occupational Characteristics,* pp. 25–78. Ann Arbor, Mich.: Institute for Social Research, University of Michigan.

Roman, P. M. 1974. "Setting for successful deviance: Drinking and deviant drinking among middle- and upper-level employees." In C. D. Bryant, ed., *Deviant Behavior: Occupational and Organizational Bases,* pp. 109–28. Chicago: Rand McNally.

Roman, R. M., and H. M. Trice. 1976. "Alcohol abuse and work organizations." In B. Kissin and H. Begleiter, eds., *The Biology of Alcoholism,* vol. 4, pp. 445–517. New York: Plenum Press.

———. 1970. "The development of deviant drinking: Occupational risk factors." *Archives of Environmental Health* 20:424–35.

———. 1968. "The sick role, labelling theory, and the deviant drinker." *International Journal of Social Psychiatry* 14:249–51.

Sadler, M., and J. E. Horst. 1972. "Company/union programs for alcoholics." *Harvard Business Review* 50 (Sept.–Oct.): 22–27, 34, 152–54.

Schmidt, W., R. G. Smart, and M. K. Moss. 1970. *Social Class and the Treatment of Alcoholism.* Addiction Research Monograph no. 7. Toronto: University of Toronto Press.

Schramm, C. J. 1977. "The development of contract language on alcohol in collective bargaining agreements." *Journal of Studies on Alcohol.* In press.

Schramm, C. J., and R. J. DeFillippi. 1975. "Characteristics of successful alcoholism treatment programs for American workers." *British Journal of Addiction to Alcohol and Other Drugs* 70:271–75.

Schramm, C. J., W. Mandell and J. Archer. 1976. *Workers Who Drink and Their Treatment in an Industrial Setting.* Final Report to the U.S. Department of Labor under U.S.D.L. Research and Development Grant no. 21-24-73-23. Baltimore: The Johns Hopkins University, School of Hygiene and Public Health.

Schur, E. M. 1971. *Labeling Deviant Behavior: Its Sociological Consequences.* New York: Harper and Row.

Seeley, J. R. 1962. "Alcoholism is a disease: Implications for social policy." In D. J.

Pittman and C. R. Snyder, eds., *Society, Culture and Drinking Patterns,* pp. 586–93. New York: Wiley and Sons.

Siassi, I., G. Crocetti, and H. R. Spiro. 1973. "Drinking patterns and alcoholism in a blue-collar population." *Quarterly Journal of Studies on Alcohol* 34:917–26.

Siegler, M., O. Humphry, and S. Newell. 1968. "Models of alcoholism." *Quarterly Journal of Studies on Alcohol* 29:571–91.

Smart, R. 1974. "Employed alcoholics treated voluntarily and under constructive coercion." *Quarterly Journal of Studies on Alcohol* 35:196–209.

Smithers Foundation. 1959. *A Company Program on Alcoholism: Basic Outline.* New York: Christopher D. Smithers Foundation.

———. 1969. *Alcoholism in Industry: Modern Procedures.* New York: Christopher D. Smithers Foundation.

———. 1970. *The Key Role of Labor in Employee Alcoholism Programs.* New York: Christopher D. Smithers Foundation.

Stamps, R. 1965. "Alcoholic employees and problem concealment." Master's thesis, Washington State University.

Sterne, M., and D. Pittman. 1965. "The concept of motivation: A source of institutional and professional blockage in the treatment of alcoholics." *Quarterly Journal of Studies on Alcohol* 26:41–57.

Stevenson, R. W. 1942. "Absenteeism in an industrial plant due to alcoholism." *Quarterly Journal of Studies on Alcohol* 2:661–68.

Straus, R. 1952. "Recognizing the problem drinker in business and industry." *Journal of Business* 25:95–100.

Straus, R., and S. D. Bacon. 1951. "Alcoholism and social stability: A study of occupational integration of 2,023 male clinic patients." *Quarterly Journal of Studies on Alcohol* 12:231–60.

Strayer, R. 1957. "A study of employment adjustment of 80 male alcoholics." *Quarterly Journal of Studies on Alcohol* 18:278–87.

Trice, H. M. 1957*a*. "Work accidents and the problem drinker: A case study." *ILR Research* 3:2–7.

———. 1957*b*. "Identifying problem drinkers on the job." *Personnel* 33:527–33.

———. 1959. *The Problem Drinker on the Job.* Bulletin 40. Ithaca: New York State School of Industrial and Labor Relations, Cornell University.

———. 1962. "The job behavior of problem drinkers." In D. J. Pittman and C. R. Snyder, eds., *Society, Culture and Drinking Patterns,* pp. 493–510. New York: Wiley.

———. 1964. "New light on identifying the alcoholic employee." *Personnel* 41:4–8.

———. 1965*a*. "Alcoholic employees: A comparison of psychotic, neurotic and 'normal' personnel." *Journal of Occupational Medicine* 7:94–99.

———. 1965*b*. "Reaction of supervisors to emotionally disturbed employees." *Journal of Occupational Medicine* 7:177–88.

Trice, H. M., and J. A. Belasco. 1966. "The alcoholic and his steward: A union problem." *Journal of Occupational Medicine* 8:481–87.

———. 1968. "Supervisory training about alcoholics and other problem employees." *Quarterly Journal of Studies on Alcohol* 29:382–98.

Trice, H. M., and P. M. Roman. 1972. *Spirits and Demons at Work: Alcohol and Other*

45646

Drugs on the Job. Ithaca. New York State School of Industrial and Labor Relations, Cornell University.

Trice, H. M., P. M. Roman, and J. A. Belasco. 1969. "Selection for treatment. A predictive evaluation of an alcoholism treatment regimen." *International Journal of the Addictions* 4:303–17.

U.S. Department of Labor. 1970. "Dealing with the drinking problem." *Manpower*, December, pp. 2–7.

Von Wiegand, R. A. 1972. "Alcoholism in industry (U.S.A.)." *British Journal of Addictions* 67:181–87.

Wanberg, K. W. 1969. "Prevalence of symptoms found among excessive drinkers." *International Journal of the Addictions* 4:169–85.

Warkov, S., S. Bacon, and A. C. Hawkins. 1965. "Social correlates of industrial problem drinking." *Quarterly Journal of Studies on Alcohol* 26:58–71.

Wellman, W. M., M. A. Maxwell, and P. O'Hollaren. 1957. "Private hospital alcoholic patients and the changing conception of the typical alcoholic." *Quarterly Journal of Studies on Alcohol* 18:388–404.

Whitehead, P. C. 1975. "The prevention of alcoholism: Divergences and convergences of two approaches." *Addictive Diseases* 1:431–43.

Williams, R. L., and G. H. Moffat, eds. 1975. *Occupational Alcoholism Programs*. Springfield, Ill.: Charles C Thomas.

Winslow, W. W., K. Hayes, L. Prentice, W. E. Powles, W. Seeman, and W. D. Ross. 1966. "Some economic estimates of job disruption from an industrial mental health project." *Archives of Environmental Health* 13:213–19.

Wrich, J. T. 1974. *The Employee Assistance Program*. Center City, Minn.: Hazelden.

TWO / The Work-Related Costs of Alcohol Abuse

RALPH E. BERRY, JR., and
JAMES P. BOLAND

A general awareness has long existed in our society that the abuse of alcohol is both pervasive and significant. Nearly everyone can recall an adverse social or personal event that could be linked to alcohol abuse. Such unpleasant events as personal degradation, broken families, accidents, acts of violence, and work not done are representative of the negative implications of alcoholism and alcohol abuse. These adverse consequences involve real losses to society in several contexts, and, of course, some of these losses represent economic costs that lend themselves to quantification. In this chapter, we are concerned with a subset of these economic costs, namely, lost production due to alcohol abuse.

The economic logic of lost production is simply that alcohol abuse may impair productivity so that less will be produced. Alcohol abuse and alcoholism can adversely affect productivity in a variety of ways and in a number of contexts. A worker's alcohol abuse can lead to absenteeism and tardiness, and when the worker is missing or late, he obviously is not contributing to production. The worker with alcohol problems is also often less productive on the job. In addition, the alcohol abuser may well have an adverse impact on his fellow workers or complementary factors of production. Certainly, overall production suffers when alcohol abuse causes capital equipment to be misused or damaged. Perhaps the most obvious case of lost production occurs when alcohol abuse causes the individual to withdraw completely or permanently from the labor force. Alcohol abuse often leads to unemployment, and sometimes to premature death.

In general, we tend to think of lost production in terms of goods and services that usually flow through the traditional market system. But individuals also

---

The work upon which this publication is based was performed in part pursuant to Contract No. HSM 42-73-114 with the National Institute on Alcohol Abuse and Alcoholism, Health Services and Mental Health Administration, Department of Health, Education, and Welfare. The authors would like to thank the Social Research Group, School of Public Health, University of California at Berkeley, for providing us with necessary unpublished data, and especially Robin Room who was of particular help.

produce goods and services in other roles as well. The family or household is the most important and obvious social system in which nonmarket production of goods and services takes place. Child care, housekeeping, meal preparation, recreation, and leisure activities are examples from an extremely long list of family-produced goods and services. When a family member has a problem with alcohol, his or her productive capacity within the family may be adversely affected, and the family will suffer the consequences. Goods and services produced by and within the household may not have market prices, but they are nonetheless valuable. Thus, to the extent that alcohol abuse lowers productivity in nonmarket activities, society also suffers a real economic loss in the form of foregone goods and services.

Since we are concerned here with the work-related costs of alcohol abuse to the economy, we will concentrate on lost production in the market sector. In fact, the task of estimating lost production in the market sector is considerably easier than in the nonmarket sector because of market prices that tend to reflect values and costs. We shall attempt an estimate of the value of lost production due to alcohol abuse which will approximate the work-related cost to the economy in the aggregate. It will also provide the basis for inferences concerning the burden that the cost places on society, firms, and individuals.

THE THEORY AND MEASUREMENT OF LOST PRODUCTION COSTS

The economic cost of lost production can be approximated by estimating the market value of what might have been produced by alcohol abusers if they had had no productivity problems associated with alcohol. Lost production attributable to alcohol abuse could be expressed in physical magnitudes, such as loaves of bread, bottles of wine, numbers of automobiles, and tons of steel. This lost output in physical terms would then have to be valued at market prices in order to allow for summation in a common unit of account. It is not feasible to measure output in physical terms for the entire economy, however, since one could hardly count the number of units not produced in all firms and organizations with alcohol-troubled workers.

An alternative measure of lost production expressed in terms such as productive man-years lost would be feasible, but the *value* of lost production would not be conveyed by such a measure. Any estimate of the value of lost production would require some estimate of the value of a man-year lost or the value of labor in production. The value of labor in production—the opportunity cost of labor—is the very information that is provided by a well-functioning market wherein the earnings of labor reflect labor's economic value in production. Hence, in order to estimate the value of lost production, a reasonably well-functioning price system is a necessary condition.

To the extent possible, we will attempt to estimate the market value of lost production by the amount of reduced earnings of workers with alcohol problems. The validity of this approach depends critically upon whether or not people are paid according to the value of their contribution to output. Technically, lost production could be valued by reduced earnings if workers were paid the value of their marginal product. The application of the economic calculus, however, does not require the strict assumption that every worker receive as earnings the value of his marginal product, but rather that there is a tendency for earnings to reflect productivity; then lost earnings will be a reasonable approximation of lost production.

A reasonable basis for estimating the cost of lost production in the market sector would be to compare the income of a representative sample of alcohol abusers with the income of a matched sample of nonabusers. If the persons in the two samples were similar in all respects except that one group included only alcohol abusers and the other included only nonabusers, then any difference in earnings would represent a reliable estimate of the impact of alcohol abuse on income. Given the prevalence of alcohol abuse, and given the reasonable assumption that earnings tend to reflect productivity, such an estimate of the impact of alcohol abuse would allow one to estimate the total cost of lost production due to alcohol abuse.

In a similar way, if one could obtain the per capita income from employment for both alcohol-abusing workers and nonabusing workers, it would be possible to generate a reasonable estimate of the total cost of lost production due to alcohol abuse. The difference in earnings between abusing and nonabusing workers would be due in part to the effect of alcohol abuse and in part to other factors which influence earnings, such as age, experience, and education. If the gross differences in earnings between abusers and nonabusers were adjusted to account for other factors known to influence earnings, the result could be taken as an estimate of the net effect of alcohol abuse on income.

In this chapter, a method similar to the latter technique will be used to estimate the cost of lost production due to alcohol abuse and alcoholism for the major component of the labor force, namely, noninstitutionalized males between the ages of 21 and 59. We were able to apply this estimation procedure because specific income and problem-drinking prevalence data were available for noninstitutionalized males between the ages of 21 and 59. Unfortunately, very little is known about either the prevalence or the economic and social behavior of other groups within society whose economic productivity may have been reduced because of alcohol abuse. In particular, prevalence and behavioral research to date has been inadequate for such groups as women, persons in institutions, and skid-row alcoholics. As a consequence, reliable estimates of the cost of lost production are most difficult to make for these groups.

Reliable cost estimation in the alcohol field depends not only on economic analysis but also on what is known about the social and economic behavior of people with alcohol problems. At present, the integration of knowledge and data from such diverse fields as alcohol research, economics, other social sciences, and health sciences is only beginning. In time, as a better understanding is gained of the role of alcohol in affecting social behavior, the scope and magnitude of the economic consequences of alcohol abuse can be estimated more precisely.

PRODUCTIVITY AND THE PREVALENCE OF ALCOHOL ABUSE

In order to estimate the value of lost production due to alcohol abuse, we need to know both the impact of alcohol abuse on productivity and the prevalence of alcohol abuse. Does the abuse of alcohol tend to lower a person's productivity? Do workers with lower productivity earn less? How many workers have alcohol problems?

Numerous studies of alcoholism within particular firms, organizations, and industries have found that workers with alcohol problems have higher average levels of absenteeism, tardiness, sickness, and the like than nonalcoholic workers (Observer and Maxwell 1959; Pell and D'Alonzo 1970, 1973; Winslow et al. 1966). Further, to the extent that virtually all such studies conclude that there are significant costs to the firm or organization, they indicate lower productivity among alcohol-abusing workers relative to the wages and salaries paid to these workers. In fact, as Trice and Roman noted in their comprehensive survey of the literature, "regardless of the method used and the dollar amounts revealed, these studies all point out that the deviant drinker costs his employer *dollars* that might be used elsewhere" (1972, p. 7).

There are some difficulties, however, with taking such indications as definite evidence of lower productivity relative to wages paid. It is quite possible that even though alcohol-abusing workers are more frequently absent, tardy, and the like, their actual wage may reflect their lower productivity. In essence, the employer may recognize that alcohol-troubled workers have lower productivity and, accordingly, pay them less than other workers. While the cost of alcohol abuse for the firm would thereby be minimized, there would be an economic cost to society in terms of lost production due to alcohol abuse, but borne by the worker, not the firm. Nevertheless, although there may be a tendency for the wages of alcohol-abusing workers to reflect their productivity, it is unlikely that the wage always measures the real value of the marginal product. A critical question is whether or not the firm is aware of a differential between what it pays (the wage) and what it gets (the dollar value of the marginal product of the worker). Even if the firm does recognize a productivity differential, it does not necessarily follow that all of it will be reflected in a wage differential. Removing the differential may well involve costs. The firm would have to expend time and resources to identify alcohol-induced lower productivity. Moreover, in many instances the firm may want to consider future as well as present productivity. Certain workers may have potentials or skills which cannot be readily replaced. Firms may choose to "invest" in some workers by paying them more than the value of their present product. A comment in a study by Observer and Maxwell (1959) illustrates the relevance of an investment view in the context of alcohol abuse: "It has been hypothesized that industry's greatest loss from problem drinking may well be the failure of certain promising young men, men with ten years and more in the company who were expected to show great talent and to assume high responsibility as they moved into their forties, but who fell (no longer 'unaccountably') by the wayside." Finally, in a complex relation between a firm and a worker organization such as a union, it just may not be worth it to try to root out the alcoholic workers or to reduce their wages to reflect the productivity difference.

To the extent that the difference in productivity due to alcohol abuse is greater than the difference in wages for whatever reason, the firm will be absorbing part of the cost of lost production. The economic cost of lost production due to alcohol abuse remains the same, but it is not borne as directly by the alcohol abuser. In fact, the firm may well be able to shift the burden to nonabusing workers in the form of lower average wages or to consumers in general in the form of higher prices for its product.

On balance, we may expect that lower productivity will be reflected by lower wages. Thus, lower earnings will be the best available approximation of lost production. In effect, since we must rely on available market information to estimate the value of lost production due to alcohol abuse, the estimate will be accurate to the extent that the market works to correct for lower productivity. In general and on average, when the market is working reasonably well, it will tend to correct for lower productivity. Still, the market does not often, if ever, work perfectly, and we would expect the correction to be less than perfect. At one extreme, if the market served to adjust each worker's wage to reflect his relative productivity exactly, an estimate of lost production generated by summing the lost earnings of alcohol abusers would result in a perfectly accurate measure. At the other extreme, if the market did not serve to adjust wages for relative productivity at all, an estimate of lost production generated by summing the lost earnings of alcohol abusers would result in a completely inaccurate estimate of zero. Hence, it might be more appropriate to note that the estimate derived is actually a measure of the lost production burden that is borne by the alcohol-abusing worker. As such, it will generally be an understatement of total lost production.

In general, the alcoholic worker has usually been identified as one whose problems are manifested through absenteeism, tardiness, sickness, and the like. Very little is known about the alcohol-troubled worker whose lower productivity is not recorded in terms of time off from the job. His problems are manifested in more subtle forms. How is the measurement problem to be coped with, given that, figuratively speaking, nearly everyone drinks? Many people drink a great deal with apparently little effect on their productivity. It might seem that one could measure income differences between abusing and nonabusing workers and consider such differences as a first approximation to the cost of alcohol abuse. But how would one determine which workers were abusers and which were nonabusers? Surely one cannot conclude that a low-income drinker has a low income because of drinking, any more than one could conclude that a high-income drinker has a high income because of drinking. If, however, one had an independent identification of alcohol-abusing workers *a priori,* one could test the hypothesis that they have lower incomes on average than their nonabusing counterparts.

The works of Cahalan and his colleagues on American drinking practices may provide a breakthrough in determining who might be classified as abusers for purposes of measuring the economic cost of alcohol abuse (Cahalan and Room 1974). They have been engaged in a longitudinal research program on the drinking practices of the general population over the past 15 years. During the course of this research they have conducted several surveys, including three national probability samples of households. These surveys have been concerned with drinking on the one hand and the consequences of drinking on the other. Thus, the respondents have been queried about problems manifested as difficulties with other people, such as spouses, relatives, friends, neighbors, co-workers, and the police. They were also asked about problems they might have handled themselves, such as financial and health problems. Cahalan and his colleagues have identified five mutually exclusive groups on the basis of individual drinking practices: (1) nondrinkers, (2) those who drink but have no problems, (3) those who drink but have potential problems only, (4) heavy drinkers with no consequences, and (5) drinkers with high consequences. The last category would appear to be the alcohol-abusing classification that is sought for our present purposes. From an economic perspective, this group is most likely to be the major source of whatever may be the economic cost of lost production due to alcohol abuse, since it consists of drinkers apparently having difficulty in their general social roles and, thus, for whom work-role problems are to be expected. The degree of the work problems of these drinkers could be measured by comparing their incomes with the incomes of nonabusers.

Empirical evidence exists that can be used to test the hypothesis that alcohol abusers (defined as drinkers with high consequences) have lower incomes than nonabusers (the first four categories in the Cahalan-Room typology). The Social Research Group, School of Public Health, University of California at Berkeley, provided us with household income data generated by their most recent national probability sample, conducted in 1969. The households are those that included a noninstitutionalized male aged 21 to 59, inclusive, in 1968. Table 2.1 outlines the income distribution of households classified according to whether or not a male alcohol abuser was present in the household. The average income of households with male abusers is, in fact, lower than the average income of households

TABLE 2.1. DISTRIBUTION OF HOUSEHOLD INCOME IN 1968 FOR HOUSEHOLDS THAT INCLUDED A NONINSTITUTIONALIZED MALE AGED 21–59

	Households with No Alcohol-Abusing Male Present		*Households with Alcohol-Abusing Male Present*		*Both Households*	
Household Income	N	%	N	%	N	%
Under $2,000	21	1.6	4	1.4	25	1.6
$2,000–$3,999	50	3.9	41	14.4	91	5.8
$4,000–$5,999	128	10.0	42	14.7	170	10.9
$6,000–$7,999	192	15.1	58	20.4	250	16.0
$8,000–$9,999	266	20.9	49	17.2	315	20.2
$10,000–$14,999	373	29.2	61	21.4	434	27.8
$15,000 and over	246	19.3	30	10.5	276	17.7
	1,276	100.0	285	100.0	1,561	100.0
Median household income	$9,861		$7,931		$9,556	
Mean household income*	$10,689		$8,725		$10,330	

SOURCE: Social Research Group, School of Public Health, University of California at Berkeley.
*Calculated by assuming $18,000 as the midpoint of the open-end income class.

with no male abusers.[1] As the table shows, there are a disproportionate number of households with male abusers present in the lowest income groups; for example, there are almost three times as many abuser as nonabuser households among the two lowest income groups. Conversely, there are proportionately fewer households with male abusers present in the highest income groups. Thus, in terms of the cumulative income distribution, for example, while slightly more than one-half of the abuser households had incomes below $8,000, less than one-third of nonabuser households had incomes below $8,000.

The household income data do not represent the earnings of individual workers, however, since they include transfer payments and such nonlabor income as interest income. The mean income data are particularly influenced by extreme observations, such as rather low incomes in the case of households that rely exclusively on transfer payments from welfare programs or rather high incomes that certain households may derive from nonlabor sources. The median income data, on the other hand, will be less influenced by nonemployment income and may reflect more closely earnings only from employment. Strictly speaking, the difference between the earnings of abusing and nonabusing workers cannot be inferred directly from these data. The findings showing that households that include male abusers have lower median earnings than those that do not, however, are consistent with the hypothesis that alcohol abusers—defined as drinkers with high consequences—have lower earnings than nonabusers. In fact, to the extent that alcohol abuse results in lower earnings due to unemployment, absenteeism, or lower wages associated with lower productivity, the lower earnings will tend to be reflected in the difference between the mean incomes of the two groups. To the extent that some part of the loss in earnings is replaced by such transfer payments as unemployment compensation or welfare payments, the actual difference in mean household income will understate the difference in earnings.

It would appear, then, that Cahalan and his colleagues have succeeded in delineating a group of drinkers who have difficulty functioning in society. It seems reasonable to deduce that this dysfunction affects their productivity and that their lowered productivity is reflected in their earnings. The deduction hinges on two assumptions: first, that a dysfunctional group has been identified, and second, that factor markets will tend to correct for the productivity implications of the dysfunction. Certainly, the income data collected by Cahalan and his colleagues tend to support this deduction. We are implicitly assuming that al-

1. The difference is statistically significant; the t-statistic for the $1,964 difference in mean household income is 6.6, which is highly significant.

cohol abuse is the cause of the dysfunction. Actually, Cahalan and his colleagues have argued only that drinking is involved and that such drinking has high consequences.

ESTIMATED PRODUCTION LOSS AMONG NONINSTITUTIONALIZED MALES AGED 21–59

While the data in Table 2.1 do indicate the extent to which alcohol abusers tend to have lower incomes than nonabusers, they do not take into account a number of additional factors known to affect income—experience, education, age, luck, intelligence, creativity, and health. One's ability to function within society might also be associated with productivity and hence, be a determinant of one's level of income. Thus, we would postulate that, other things being equal, alcohol abuse will lower productivity and be reflected in lower earnings. If the income data summarized in Table 2.1 are to be used to estimate lost production due to alcohol abuse, some account must be taken of and an appropriate adjustment made for the likelihood that other things are not equal. If such an adjustment were made for any differences between the abusing and nonabusing groups with respect to other factors that affect income, the net difference between the average annual earnings of the two groups would be a reasonable basis for estimating the cost of lost production due to alcohol abuse.

Unfortunately, the data provided by the Social Research Group at Berkeley are such that only age differences can be adjusted for directly. The average household incomes in 1968 by age of noninstitutionalized males included in the household are outlined in Table 2.2. In fact, analysis of the data in Table 2.2 indicates that some 9.3 percent of the gross difference in mean household income is due to age differences between the two groups. Thus, approximately $183 of the $1,964 difference in mean income between households with and without alcohol-abusing males can be accounted for by age differences between the two groups.

Although age is undoubtedly correlated with other factors that affect income (such as experience), an additional adjustment would be desirable to account for factors that affect income but that are not correlated with age.[2] What is needed is an adjustment factor to apply to the gross difference in income between the abusing and nonabusing groups that will serve to net out the part of the difference due to factors other than alcohol abuse that are known to influence income. In a

2. Of course, since age "picks up" the influence of factors correlated with age, an adjustment of 9.3 percent for age would account for more than just the net age effect.

TABLE 2.2 ANNUAL AVERAGE HOUSEHOLD INCOME IN 1968 OF NONINSTITUTIONALIZED MALES INCLUDED IN THE HOUSEHOLD, BY AGE

	Number of Households			Mean Household Income			Median Household Income		
Age Group	*Without Alcohol Abuser*	*With Alcohol Abuser*	*Total*	*Without Alcohol Abuser*	*With Alcohol Abuser*	*Difference*	*Without Alcohol Abuser*	*With Alcohol Abuser*	*Difference*
21–29	284	108	392	$ 9,692	$7,875	$1,817	$ 8,857	$7,121	$1,736
30–39	330	66	396	11,252	9,303	1,949	10,808	8,857	1,951
40–49	331	59	390	11,118	8,983	2,135	10,026	7,934	2,092
50–59	331	52	383	10,556	9,462	1,094	10,023	8,756	1,267
All Ages	1,276	285	1,561	10,689	8,725	1,964	9,861	7,931	1,930

SOURCE: Social Research Group, School of Public Health, University of California at Berkeley.

recently published comprehensive study, Luft (1975) utilized such an approach to measure the impact of poor health on earnings. His empirical results provide the basis for the adjustment factor we need. Using data from the 1967 Survey of Economic Opportunity, a national sample of all adults aged 18 to 64, Luft calculated the mean annual earnings of sick and well workers for the year 1966. As one would expect, the earnings of those in good health were considerably higher than the earnings of those in poor health. By means of multiple regression, Luft was able to analyze the gross differences and determine the net effect of poor health on earnings. In effect, his analysis took into account several socioeconomic factors, such as age, education, and family structure. Even after controlling for these factors, Luft found a net difference between the annual earnings of those in good and poor health, although the net difference, of course, was somewhat lower. Of particular interest, however, is the estimate Luft derived of the proportion of the gross difference between the groups in male earnings that is accounted for by socioeconomic factors. In fact, such factors accounted for 23.9 percent of the gross difference. Thus, we might take an additional adjustment of some 14.6 percent (23.9 − 9.3) to account for factors other than age that affect differences in mean income between the abusing and nonabusing groups. Alternatively, we could take an adjustment of 23.9 percent of the gross difference.

The gross adjustment suggested by the Luft study seems a reasonable approximation of socioeconomic influences for a number of reasons. First, the data available for alcohol abusers indicates that age-related factors account for 9.3 percent of the gross difference. Second, both the Social Research Group data and the Luft data came from national probability samples, and hence, statistically, the two samples would be expected to have similar socioeconomic characteristics in the aggregate. Although the Social Research Group sample was partitioned by alcohol abuse and the Luft sample was partitioned by health status, to the extent that alcohol abuse is a disease, one might expect the characteristics of the relevant subsamples to be somewhat similar. Finally, even if the adjustment is but an approximation, it serves to avoid overstating the net effect of alcohol abuse on earnings.

Given the data made available by the Social Research Group and the adjustment factor suggested by Luft's study, we now have sufficient data to generate an estimate of the economic cost of lost production due to alcohol abuse among noninstitutionalized males between the ages of 21 and 59. An estimate of lower earnings due to alcohol abuse by age is outlined in Table 2.3. The total number of households including a male as reported by the Bureau of the Census for 1970 is shown in column 1. The prevalence data in column 2 are derived from Table 2.2

TABLE 2.3. AN ESTIMATE OF THE LOWER EARNINGS OF HOUSEHOLDS WITH AN ALCOHOL-ABUSING MALE PRESENT

Age Group	*All Households Including a Male* (N)	*Households with Male Abuser Present* (%)	*Estimated Number of Households with Male Abuser Present* (N)	*Estimated Net Difference in Mean Household Income* ($)	*Estimated Lower Earnings due to Alcohol Abuse* (Millions of $)
21–29	7,012	27.6	1,935.3	1,524	2,949.4
30–39	10,156	16.7	1,696.1	1,635	2,773.1
40–49	10,851	15.1	1,638.5	1,791	2,934.6
50–59	9,553	13.6	1,299.2	918	1,192.7
All Ages	37,572		6,569.1		9,849.8

SOURCES: The total number of households including a male is from U.S. Bureau of the Census, *Family Composition, 1970: Subject Report* (Washington, D.C.: U.S. Government Printing Office, 1973). The percentage of households with male abuser present was derived from data in Table 2.2. The estimated net difference in mean household income was derived by adjusting the differences in Table 2.2 (see text).

and represent the proportion of households with a male abuser present. Column 4 gives the estimated net differences in mean household income adjusted to account for other socioeconomic factors that affect earnings. The estimated net differences in household income shown in column 5 serve as a reasonable approximation of the effect of alcohol abuse on earnings. Since the income data were for 1968 and the number of households for 1970, we are actually either overstating the amount for 1968 or understating the amount for 1970. However, since we are not trying to generate a specific amount for a given year, the approximation is a useful one for present purposes. More than 6.5 million households included a male alcohol abuser between the ages of 21 and 59. In the aggregate, households with an alcohol-abusing male present had lower earnings due to alcohol abuse on the order of $9.8 billion. In fact, they actually had lower earnings of almost $13 billion, but socioeconomic factors accounted for 23.9 percent of their lower earnings.

If careful consideration is given to the several obvious ways in which this surrogate may be a biased estimate, it would seem that $9.8 billion does indeed represent a reasonably conservative estimate of the economic cost of lost production due to alcohol abuse among noninstitutionalized males between the ages of 21 and 59. First, we have not taken the gross difference in income between abuser and nonabuser households as a measure of the difference in earnings due to alcohol abuse. Rather, we have attempted to adjust the difference to account for the other factors—such as age, education, and family structure—that undoubtedly influence earnings. Clearly, the gross difference in mean income between abuser and nonabuser households represents more than the net effect of alcohol abuse. By adjusting the difference to account for other factors, we have avoided an obvious overstatement of the net loss due to alcohol abuse. Moreover, to the extent that lower earnings of abusers were offset in part by transfer payments, such as unemployment compensation or welfare payments, the difference in average income between abuser and nonabuser households would understate the loss due to alcohol abuse. Similarly, to the extent that other household members moved into the labor force in order to cushion the loss of earnings, the difference in average income between abuser and nonabuser households would understate the loss due to alcohol abuse.[3] Furthermore, the age distribution was truncated at both ends. No amount is included in the estimate for alcohol-abusing workers below the age of 21 or over the age of 59. Finally, no amount is included in the estimate for working women who were alcohol abusers. While, on balance, $9.8 billion would seem to be a conservative estimate of the economic cost of lost production among the civilian labor force, it is a better approximation of the economic cost of lost production in the market sector than previously available data allowed.

THE BURDEN OF PRODUCTION LOST TO ALCOHOL ABUSE

We have estimated that alcohol-abusing workers earn almost $10 billion less in the aggregate than they would if they were not abusers. Clearly, this represents a significant economic cost. In fact, as noted previously, the estimate derived is actually a measure of the lost production burden that is borne by the alcohol-abusing worker. As such, it is undoubtedly an understatement of total lost production. There is no empirical basis for refining this estimate, but we can indicate the ways in which some part of the burden may be shared with nonabusers and thereby gain some insight into the potential magnitude of the problem.

As discussed earlier in this chapter, it is likely that not all of the adverse impact

3. For example, if alcohol abuse caused a husband's earnings to fall by $5,000, but his wife took a part-time job and earned $3,000 to help maintain the household's standard of living, the gross difference in household income would appear to be only $2,000 less, but that understates the loss due to alcohol abuse by $3,000. The discerning reader will recognize that the lost production in the market sector has been lowered at the expense of lost production in the nonmarket sector.

of alcohol abuse on productivity is reflected in the earnings of abusing workers, since employers may not adjust wages to reflect lower productivity. To the extent that this is true, the burden borne by the abusing worker is less than the total loss of production due to alcohol abuse. When the firm absorbs part of the cost of lost production, the ultimate burden may be borne by the firm in the form of lower profits, by nonabusing workers in the form of lower wages, or by consumers in the form of higher prices for the firm's product. In the case of governmental organizations, the ultimate burden may be borne by taxpayers. Clearly, the market structure within which the firm operates will have something to do with the relative shares of the burden of lost production. In more competitive markets, one would expect the share borne by the alcohol-abusing worker to be somewhat greater. In labor markets characterized by collective bargaining for wages, a greater proportion of the burden may be shifted to nonabusing workers. In less competitive markets, more of the burden might be shifted to consumers in the form of higher prices; in the public sector, to taxpayers in the form of higher taxes. Although we have no basis for even speculating on the magnitude of this additional burden, it clearly represents the potential for a significant additional economic cost. Even if abusers themselves absorb 90 percent of the burden, others would suffer a loss on the order of $1 billion.

The work-related cost of alcohol abuse has further ramifications as well. Lost production usually results in lost income. In the absence of any social response to this loss, the burden would be borne in large part by individual alcohol abusers and their families, with some part shifted to the firm, other workers, and consumers. But society in general has been unwilling to ignore the plight of families and individuals having especially low incomes: rather, the social welfare system has evolved as a response to categorical misfortune. Of course, the social welfare system does not exist because of alcohol abuse, but some part of the client load and some part of the cost of the system does represent a response to alcohol abuse as one kind of personal and family misfortune. If alcohol abuse did not exist, then society could either spend less on its social welfare system or provide more services to those whose misfortune is not associated with alcohol abuse. Indeed, alcohol abuse undoubtedly affects such programs as unemployment compensation, workmen's compensation, and public assistance for low-income families and individuals. To the extent that alcohol-abusing workers have higher unemployment rates, higher accident rates, and lower incomes in general, they are costly to firms and other taxpayers, who must pay higher unemployment taxes, higher insurance premiums, and higher taxes in general. Certainly, these work-related costs of alcohol abuse are not insignificant.

REFERENCES

Berry, R. E., Jr., and J. P. Boland. Forthcoming. *The Economic Cost of Alcohol Abuse*. New York: The Free Press.

Cahalan, D., and R. Room. 1974. *Problem Drinking among American Men*. New Brunswick, N.J.: Rutgers Center of Alcohol Studies.

Luft, H. S. 1975. "The impact of poor health on earnings." *Review of Economics and Statistics* 57:43–57.

Observer and M. A. Maxwell. 1959. "A study of absenteeism, accidents and sickness payments in problem drinkers in one industry." *Quarterly Journal of Studies on Alcohol* 20:302–12.

Pell, S., and C. A. D'Alonzo. 1970. "Sickness absenteeism of alcoholics." *Journal of Occupational Medicine* 12:198–210.

———. 1973. "A five-year mortality study of alcoholics." *Journal of Occupational Medicine* 15:120–25.

Trice, H. M., and P. M. Roman. 1972. *Spirits and Demons at Work: Alcohol and Other Drugs on the Job*. Ithaca: New York State School of Industrial and Labor Relations, Cornell University.

Winslow, W. W., K. Hayes, L. Prentice, W. E. Powles, W. Seeman, and W. D. Ross. 1966. "Some economic estimates of job disruption." *Archives of Environmental Health* 13:213–19.

THREE / Differential Use of an Alcoholism Policy in Federal Organizations by Skill Level of Employees

HARRISON M. TRICE and
JANICE M. BEYER

Like the larger American society within which they are embedded, formal work organizations inevitably have a system of social stratification consisting of a hierarchy of positions—statuses that are unequal in power, income, prestige, and psychic gratification. Furthermore, in American society, these work-world positions are the most important source of general social status (Bendix and Lipset 1966; Tumin 1967). Within work organizations, status hierarchies become operative through occupations and associated skill levels. Occupations vary widely in terms of the power, authority, and responsibility they yield in an organization's structure. They differ in the prestige they bring to the jobholder from the broader community. Quite obviously, they differ in the degree of psychic income they provide. For those without an occupational identity and commitment, the work organization typically provides status by means of assigned skill levels that function in status terms as occupations. In sum, the work place generally functions largely through a status hierarchy.

THE HYPOTHESIS

In this chapter we examine how this status system influences the implementation of a formal alcoholism policy in a sample of 71 federal civil service installations in the northeastern United States. Our general hypothesis was that adoption and use of the legally mandated policy would be significantly greater when applied to

---

The authors wish gratefully to acknowledge grant 1 R01 AA2989-01 from the National Institute on Alcohol Abuse and Alcoholism, which provided funds for the research reported here.

relatively low-status, low-skilled employees as compared with higher status levels of employees. The hypothesis was derived from three sources. First, two earlier studies of single companies found status-related differences in the identification and treatment of problem drinkers. In the first study, Warkov et al. (1965) asked supervisors in a large utility with no formal alcoholism policy to identify the problem drinkers in a sample of employees under their supervision. They secured these identifications through the mail. They concluded: "Incidence of identification as a problem drinker varied inversely with social, occupational, and organizational status of employees" (p. 70). However, they cautioned about concluding that the 62 out of 5,479 employees identified as problem drinkers constituted a total count. Rather, they put their data in terms of the "risk of identification as a problem drinker," clearly indicating that they believed that their data represented a screening process in which supervisors may identify drinkers differentially on the basis of occupational or skill level status (p. 69). The second study (Trice 1965*a*, 1965*b*) was conducted in a large utility company that had had a formal alcoholism policy for nine years. The status levels of employees processed under the company's alcoholism program were compared with samples of "normal" employees and with samples of employees who had been diagnosed as neurotic or psychotic. Trice concluded: "In social status terms, diagnosed alcoholics were found in low status job situations: less pay, fewer promotions, more dependents, less education, blue-collar jobs of a manual nature, requiring mobility rather than a fixed position. All these suggest rather low job prestige. But these data mirror diagnosed alcoholics only. The diagnostic and program process may be selective" (1965*a*, p. 95).

Second, our observations of policies and programs in actual operation in specific corporations, companies, and unions over a period of several years have been consistent with the hypothesis (Trice 1966). Over and over we have heard union officials criticize an alcoholism policy because it was applied, often both in theory and in practice, only to employees in the bargaining unit. When we used observation as a research method or used an anthropological approach, we arrived at a similar hunch in other research settings—namely, that high status, elite alcoholics existed, but that they were so shielded by various factors that a policy never became sufficiently operative to cover them (Trice and Belasco 1970).

Third, various deductions led us to this hypothesis. When we systematically considered the issue of which factors might lead to differential application of an alcoholism policy according to the skill level of the employees involved, several logical arguments emerged: (1) Lower-status persons may, in fact, have more drinking problems (Cahalan 1970) and (2) may be less motivated and less effective in covering them up. (3) The performance of lower-status employees is probably much more visible to supervisors than that of higher-status employees. Lower-status employees often punch time clocks and work in open spaces rather than in private offices. (4) Additionally, work supervisors of high-status employees probably maintain less social distance between themselves and their subordinates than do supervisors of lower-status subordinates. Thus, the identification of such a subordinate as a problem drinker may spill over into social life and also may be personally threatening to the supervisor, who sees himself as generally similar to that employee. Professional workers, especially, would tend to be seen as more similar to the supervisor himself than would relatively unskilled employees. (5) The use of an alcoholism policy with a highly skilled or professional employee may seem to carry substantially higher risks for a supervisor than if he used the policy on low-status subordinates. Such an employee may be more effective and articulate in his own defense, which will probably include resentment against the supervisor. Moreover, bad performance may be seen as reflecting back on the supervisor and his unit. (6) Some employees at higher skill levels may hold jobs in which there would be substantial risks associated with defective job performance, including alcohol-related deficiencies. Such jobs or occupations include those that interface with powerful client or adversary groups, or that involve substantial levels of responsibility for public welfare. Because of these risks, employees with drinking problems may themselves leave such jobs, or—more likely—they may be weeded out of these jobs by supervisors in ways not connected with a formal alcoholism policy.

This hypothesis was tested as part of a larger study of the implementation of the federal civil service alcoholism policy and program. This alcoholism policy was mandated through legislation passed by Congress in 1970—Public Law 91-616, the so-called Hughes Act. This law provided for the development and maintenance of programs and services designed to deal with prevention and treatment of alcoholism and alcohol abuse among federal civilian employees and with their rehabilitation. Subsequently, in the summer of 1971, the Civil Service Commission issued a formal policy statement (FPML 792-4) that instructed the heads of the various departments and agencies within the federal government to issue internal implementing instructions relative to the new alcoholism policy by 1 December 1971.

The Cornell Program on Occupational Health and Alcoholism began to collect historical data and background information relative to the federal alcoholism policy in the winter of 1972/73. The major data collection effort, however, occurred within the federal installations for which this policy was formulated and within which this policy was supposed to be implemented. These installations provide an excellent setting in which to test our hypothesis about status and the differential use of an alcoholism policy, because they include diverse occupations and technologies. Our sample included installations within nine major executive branches of the federal government: Agriculture; Commerce; General Services Administration; Health, Education, and Welfare (HEW); Housing and Urban Development (HUD); Interior; Justice; Transportation; and Treasury. Data were collected within these agencies beginning in the late spring of 1974, providing a three-year interval between the promulgation of the policy and our efforts to assess its actual implementation.

SAMPLING AND RESEARCH METHODS

In order to give the results of our study the maximum generalizability, we decided to sample as inclusively as was possible and practical from among the federal installations in which civilian employees worked. We therefore obtained a list of all the nonmilitary, inspectable units of the Boston, Philadelphia, and New York regions under the jurisdiction of the Federal Civil Service Commission. The sample was restricted to the northeastern region in order to keep travel time and expense within reasonable bounds.[1] Agencies involved in covert operations (e.g., CIA, FBI) were eliminated because of practical difficulties of eliciting cooperation and contacting random samples from the population of supervisors. Finally, installations with fewer than 50 employees were eliminated. Once the list had been modified in terms of these three restrictions, it served as the sampling frame or population for a two-stage sampling procedure.

First, a stratified, random sample of installations was drawn, with strata determined by installation size (small, fewer than 150 employees; large, more than this number), the nine executive departments, and the three civil service regions. Because of the distribution of the stratified characteristics in the population, we were unable to fill all 54 cells of this design with two installations, but we maintained the sampling design whenever possible to yield a final sample of 71 installations. The second stage of sampling occurred within each of these installations when a systematic sample of supervisors was drawn from within the installation, with the size of the sample inversely proportional to the size of the installation. This resulted in a sample size of 651 supervisors.[2] Different research instruments were designed for supervisors, directors (heads of installations), and

1. Professor Paul Roman of Tulane University carried out a parallel study in the southern civil service regions.

2. Both samples were substantially sustained: only one installation declined cooperation and had to be replaced; six supervisors refused and were replaced. Changes in the number of employees within installations is continual, and some of these changes are substantial in magnitude. Despite continual checking and revision of the sample list and sample, two installations with fewer than 50 employees ended up in the final sample and data collection effort.

the alcoholism coordinator—a role especially designated in the formal policy. The instruments were a combination of questionnaire and interview items, including a wide variety of data generating techniques aimed at measuring the extent of actual, projected, and expected use of the alcoholism policy. These included self-reported behaviors, perceptions, and attitudes measured by Likert scales, semantic differentials, and behavioral vignettes. A wide variety of data was also collected on independent variables which we expected to be associated with policy implementation. Each interview-questionnaire was administered face-to-face by a trained field interviewer in a private location, typically the respondent's office. Since samples of supervisors were not drawn until we actually reached a sample installation, no supervisors knew in advance that they were to be interviewed. In only a few of the largest installations did interviewing by our teams take more than one day to complete. The opportunities for discussion among respondents were thus minimized, and we also asked them not to discuss the interviews.

In these interviews, we asked all supervisors to describe in detail the kind of work done by employees under their supervision. From these descriptions, we created a quasi-scale that classified supervisors on the basis of the types of employees they supervised into the following categories: (1) unskilled only; (2) unskilled and skilled; (3) skilled only; (4) unskilled, skilled, and professional; (5) skilled and professional; and (6) professional only.[3] The assumption behind this scale was that increasing values represent higher levels of skill and occupational status within the group of employees supervised by a given supervisor.

For the analysis reported here, our dependent variables included items designed to indicate the degree of diffusion of information about the policy, supervisors' familiarity with an assessment of the policy, actual occasions to use the policy, and projected use of the policy—i.e., how a supervisor would act in a specific but hypothetical situation involving the alcoholism policy in a behavioral vignette. Since both the skill-level scale and most of the implementation items were ordinal scales, we decided to use chi-square tests and, when appropriate,

3. Employees were considered professional if they worked in a defined occupation that usually required at least a bachelor's degree for entry and for which occupational skills, status, and even job titles tend to be transferable from one employer to another, whether in or out of the federal service. Examples are accountants, lawyers, chemists, nurses, etc. Employees were considered skilled if they worked at a job that required specific skills that could not be acquired in relatively rapid training programs. Examples are secretaries, claims adjusters, plumbers, lower-level computer personnel, etc. Employees were considered unskilled if their work did not require much training. Examples are janitors, warehousemen, bottle washers in laboratories, gate keepers, receptionists, switchboard operators, etc.

one-way analyses of variance to determine whether there was differential diffusion, familiarity, acceptance, and use of the policy at lower as compared with higher skill levels.

A second source of data to test the hypothesis was available from alcoholism coordinators. Since there was only one coordinator representing each installation, we had to devise a way to describe the distributions of skill levels within an entire installation. In order to characterize the skill level of a given installation, the proportion of supervisor respondents who reported having unskilled, skilled, and/or professional employees under their supervision was calculated. Installations were then divided into low, medium, and high groupings within each skill category, assigning installations to these categories so that each category would represent as close to one-third of the installations as ties permitted. This information on the relative proportion of skill levels supervised within each installation was then analyzed against data obtained from the alcoholism coordinator of that installation.

RESULTS: THE SUPERVISOR

Throughout the results of the analysis of the supervisory data, the patterning of statistically significant results was surprisingly consistent and generally in support of our hypothesis.[4] Larger numbers of supervisors with only unskilled employees reported that they were more familiar with various provisions of the alcohol policy than did supervisors with more skilled employees. Those supervisors with mixtures of all three types of employees and those with all professionals were least likely to claim much familiarity with policy provisions. Supervisors of the unskilled only were significantly more familiar with provisions for leave ($X^2 = 25.12$, 12*df*, $p = .014$), union relations ($X^2 = 34.73$, 12*df*, $p = .0005$), and reporting provisions ($X^2 = 33.08$, 12*df*, $p = .0009$). Moreover, in contrast to those with higher-status employees, they believed that the policy represented an important step for the federal government to take ($X^2 = 35.74$, 12*df*, $p = .0076$). Additionally, when asked how much training they had received in the alcoholism policy, the supervisors of the less-skilled employees reported more hours spent learning about the policy than did supervisors at higher skill levels. Taken together, these three findings clearly suggest that supervisors of relatively lower skill levels of employees were more familiar with and more

4. Unless reported, results were significant at $p = .05$. The data reported here are the first to be published from this study, and these may be modified somewhat and clarified further as the results of multivariate and other more sophisticated analyses become available from subsequent work.

favorable in their assessment of the federal alcoholism policy. They were proponents of the policy and better informed about it.

Under such conditions, we expected that a significantly higher percentage of such supervisors would report that they had used the alcoholism policy. As shown in Table 3.1, this was indeed the case. When we asked supervisors if they had had an opportunity to use the alcohol policy, eleven percent of the total reported some occasion to do so. This probably means they had had some employee under their supervision whom they thought might have a drinking problem. This proportion, however, jumped to 30 percent for supervisors who had only unskilled subordinates and fell to 0 percent for supervisors having only professional employees. Thus, we found that supervisors of relatively unskilled employees were not only better informed about and proponents of the alcoholism policy, but they were actually more likely to encounter and recognize occasions to use that policy (Table 3.1).

Other significant differences reinforce these findings. Among the different types of supervisors, those of unskilled employees were most likely to report that they either had taken negative actions, such as official reprimands or other disciplinary actions, against the problem drinker or else had done nothing at all about the situation. Their problem-drinking employees, by their account, were also least likely to be referred for medical or other appropriate help (Table 3.2). While the problem drinker was discharged in about 10 percent of the cases handled by supervisors of unskilled, or a mixture of unskilled and skilled, employees, no firings took place at higher skill levels. However, an equal proportion of the higher status problem-drinking employees (10 percent) were trans-

TABLE 3.1 PERCENTAGE OF SUPERVISORS WHO HAVE USED THE ALCOHOLISM POLICY, BY SKILL LEVEL OF EMPLOYEES SUPERVISED

Used Alcohol Policy	*Skill Level of Employees Supervised*						
	Unskilled Only	*Unskilled and Skilled*	*Skilled Only*	*Unskilled and Skilled Professional*	*Skilled and Professional*	*Professional Only*	*All Skill Levels*
	(N=34)	(N=84)	(N=239)	(N=11)	(N=242)	(N=16)	(N=626)
No	70.6	90.5	88.7	90.9	90.1	100.0	88.8
Yes	29.4	9.5	11.3	9.1	9.9	0.0	11.2
	100.0	100.0	100.0	100.0	100.0	100.0	100.0

$X^2 = 14.06$, $5df$, $p < .02$

TABLE 3.2 PERCENTAGES OF SUPERVISORS TAKING VARIOUS ACTIONS TO DEAL WITH ALCOHOL PROBLEM, BY SKILL LEVEL OF EMPLOYEES SUPERVISED

	Skill Level of Employees Supervised			
	*Some Unskilled**	*Skilled Only*	*Some Professional**	*All Levels*
Types of Action	(N=22)	(N=33)	(N=33)	(N=88)
Failed to help employee†	36.0	18.0	9.0	19.0
Referred employee elsewhere in organization	18.0	6.0	18.0	14.0
Counseled employee	32.0	33.0	36.0	34.0
Referred employee for help‡	14.0	42.0	36.0	33.0
	100.0	99.0	99.0	100.0

$X^2 = 10.89$, $6df$, $p < .10$

*Combined categories to meet chi-square requirements for all sizes.
†Either took action detrimental to employee or no action.
‡Referred to alcohol coordinator, medical resources, or other helping resources.

ferred. No transfers occurred with supervisors of lower skill levels. Taken together, these data suggest that supervisors at higher skill levels could more readily send their problem-drinking employees elsewhere within the organization, while supervisors of unskilled employees may have been limited to terminating such employees because their transferability was less.

Since most supervisors do not have occasion to use the alcoholism policy, we also asked our sample of supervisors how they would behave in certain hypothetical situations relevant to the alcoholism policy (the behavioral vignettes mentioned earlier). Some of these results were surprising. For example, when we asked supervisors what they would do about an employee who was increasingly absent, only 25 percent gave the answer called for in the policy, namely to refer the employee for official counseling (Table 3.3). Supervisors with skilled and professional employees were significantly more likely to opt for managing the problem between themselves and the employee. More than 60 percent of such supervisors selected this action, which is clearly not what is intended by the alcoholism policy, even though they knew we were studying the implementation of that policy. By contrast, 40 to 50 percent of supervisors of the two lower skill levels chose this option. The latter, in turn, were significantly more likely to

TABLE 3.3 PERCENTAGES OF SUPERVISORS WHO WOULD TAKE OFFICIAL ACTION AGAINST AN EMPLOYEE WHO IS INCREASINGLY ABSENT, BY SKILL LEVEL OF EMPLOYEES SUPERVISED

	Skill Level of Employees Supervised				
Choice of Action	*Unskilled*	*Unskilled and Skilled*	*Skilled*	*Some Professionals*	*All Levels*
Officially reprimand	21.0	30.0	16.0	12.0	16.0
Officially suggest counseling	29.0	30.0	24.0	24.0	25.0
Manage between ourselves	50.0	40.0	61.0	64.0	59.0
	100.0	100.0	101.0	100.0	100.0

$X^2 = 24.11$, $6df$, $p < .001$

report that they would issue an official reprimand to a chronic absentee: from 20 to 30 percent of them chose this option—nearly twice the proportion of supervisors of higher skill levels.

RESULTS: THE ALCOHOLISM COORDINATOR

If our findings for the supervisor are correct, the reactions and behaviors of the alcoholism coordinator should be consistent with them, even though coordinators perform different functions vis-à-vis the policy. With this in mind, we analyzed various policy implementation measures from the coordinators' responses by skill level.[5] Recall that the skill level of the employees within an installation served by a given coordinator was characterized by computing the proportion of supervisors who reported any subordinates at that skill level and then using that proportion to characterize that skill level for that installation. For example, if six out of eight supervisors reported some professional employees under their supervision, then the proportion for "professional skill level" for that installation would be 75 percent, and it would rank toward the top or high end of the installations for the professional skill level. These proportions were ranked, and the ranks were divided into as equal as possible groups, given the ties in the rankings. This means that, for this analysis, installation skill levels are labelled "high," "medium," or "low" only in a sense relative to the remaining installa-

5. Some coordinators in our sample served more than one installation. In these results, the data of such coordinators are considered only once, usually for the installation where they worked. Being an alcoholism coordinator is usually only part of that person's duties. Therefore, $n = 64$ for these analyses.

tions in our sample. The results of our analysis by proportions of the three skill levels follow.

Installations with a low proportion of skilled employees were most likely to have a staff to assist the coordinator in implementing the alcohol policy (X^2 = 6.398, *2df*, p = < .04). Referral to community agencies was also related to skill level (X^2 = 5.798, *2df*, p = < .05). Installations with high proportions of unskilled employees, low proportions of skilled employees, and/or low proportions of professional employees were most likely to refer employees to community agencies. Such installations, through their coordinators, also more often referred problem drinkers to counselors (X^2 = 8.17, *2df*, p = < .017), more frequently used disciplinary action (X^2 = 5.28, *2df*, p = < .07), more frequently confered with the problem drinker's supervisor (X^2 = 4.897, *2df*, p = < .09), and generally reported more occasions to use the policy. This means that the coordinators' greatest use of the policy during the previous year (mid-1973 to mid-1974) had occurred in installations with high proportions of unskilled employees; that is, the number of employees who had actually been handled under the provisions of the alcoholism policy was significantly greater where the proportions of supervisors of unskilled employees was high. This is consistent with another finding that coordinators at installations with few skilled workers were most likely to believe that there were employees in their installation who could benefit from the alcoholism policy.

At this point we became interested in whether or not the coordinator's being officially appointed by the director would matter, as opposed to coordinators who reported acting "unofficially" in that capacity. Where the proportion of skilled employees was low and the coordinator saw himself as "official," the number of cases to which that coordinator applied the policy was significantly greater (11.6 versus 3.0 and 1.2 where proportions of skilled workers were medium and high, respectively). This did not occur at any other skill level, regardless of the official or unofficial status of the coordinator.

Both supervisors and alcohol coordinators were asked whether or not they agreed with specific statements in accord with the intent of the alcoholism policy and with other statements that were less in agreement with the policy's intent (Table 3.4). Coordinators in installations with higher proportions of unskilled employees or low proportions of professional employees were more likely than other coordinators to endorse the statement that a supervisor should counsel an employee who appeals to him about a drinking problem (p < .10), and in this regard, they were in agreement with the policy. The coordinators in installations with many unskilled workers also more often endorsed a definition of alcoholism that was in accord with the policy. However, coordinators with low proportions

TABLE 3.4 RESULTS OF ANALYSES OF VARIANCE ON AGREEMENT WITH AND DIFFUSION OF INFORMATION ON THE ALCOHOL POLICY BY ALCOHOL COORDINATORS, CONTROLLING FOR SKILL LEVELS OF EMPLOYEES

		Alcohol Coordinators (Mean)			
		*Agreement**			
Variable	*Skill Level of Employees*	*Low*	*Medium*	*High*	*p*†
Supervisor should counsel if employee asks about problem	Unskilled	4.429	3.957	5.263	.10
A person is an alcoholic if his drinking causes a problem with health, relationships, or finances.	Unskilled	4.667	5.130	5.362	.05
	Professional	5.571	4.684	5.087	.05
Supervisor should try to identify alcohol problems before job affected	Professional	5.143	5.474	4.429	.10
Alcoholism is a treatable illness	Skilled	5.083	5.769	5.711	.05
		Diffusion			
		Low	*Medium*	*High*	*p*†
Forms of information given union on alcohol policy	Skilled	1.750	0.769	0.825	.05
Sources of information on alcohol policy given to employees	Skilled	1.917	0.769	1.150	.10
Number of sources from which coordinator received information	Skilled	1.750	0.692	1.025	.10
When appointed alcohol coordinator‡	Professional	3.050	4.000	2.714	.05

*High = agree (6-point scale ranging from 1 = disagree strongly to 6 = agree strongly).
†As determined by *F*-tests of one-way analysis of variance.
‡Low = recent appointment.

of professional employees were also most likely to endorse the statement that they should try to identify drinking problems before job performance is affected ($p < .10$)—a step that exceeds the intent of the federal policy, which urges supervisors to concentrate on job performance as the criterion for intervention. Also, coordinators with low proportions of skilled employees were least likely to agree that alcoholism is a treatable illness—certainly a statement that the federal alcoholism policy was intended to endorse.

Consistent with the data on supervisors' familiarity with policy provisions, the coordinators serving lower skill levels reported significantly more forms of information on the alcoholism policy given to unions and that rank-and-file employees were informed about the policy from a greater number of different sources than in other installations (Table 3.4). Furthermore, these coordinators themselves had received information regarding provisions of the policy from significantly more sources. A related finding was that where the proportion of professional employees was high, coordinators clearly tended to be appointed at a later date. These coordinators, in turn, were least likely to believe that there were employees in their organization who could benefit from the policy.

Still other status differences emerged. Coordinators in installations with higher proportions of professional employees reported better medical facilities.[6] Perhaps this is one reason why they were more likely to use medical evidence in deciding whether or not a given problem was an alcohol problem, whereas coordinators in places with more unskilled employees were more likely than other coordinators to use observations of behavior to make that decision. Either employees with lower skill levels were more likely to exhibit behavior that was obviously tied to drinking, or coordinators were more likely to consider problem behavior evidence of drinking among lower-level employees.

The major criterion specified by the policy for deciding that an employee might be referred for counseling and other action by the alcohol coordinator is the question of work performance. Poor performance, including absenteeism and tardiness, is considered sufficient reason for a supervisor to refer an employee for consideration under the alcoholism policy. This is especially true where work performance has been declining or fluctuating. While all coordinators reported that this was the main reason for deciding that an employee had an alcohol problem, with increasing proportions of unskilled employees the frequency of use of this criterion declined from 44 percent to 28 percent, while the frequency of using other observed behavior increased from 12 percent to 24 percent.

Since these data and those from the supervisors strongly suggest that policy implementation was much more vigorous where the mix of job skill levels was toward lower-status jobs, we decided to analyze data from coordinators on the *frequency* (estimates of number of times used) with which they used specific

6. Medical department available: $X^2 = 5.5$, $2df$, $p = <.06$; provisions for medical services available in absence of medical department: $X^2 = 10.29$, $4df$, $p = <.037$.

policy procedures. If these data also showed that policy use was more frequent at the lower skill levels, our hypothesis would be further supported. This, in fact, happened; the results again exhibited a pattern consistent with the findings from the data from supervisors. Where there were low proportions of skilled employees, medical benefits and community agencies were most frequently used, and disciplinary procedures and referral to counselors within the agency were also more frequently used. The use of union contacts, however, was highest in installations with medium proportions of skilled workers.

Finally, coordinators with high proportions of unskilled employees were significantly more likely to feel that they needed additional information on how to implement the alcoholism policy ($X^2 = 5.78$, $2df$, $p < .055$), and how to prepare statistical reports on the policy for the installation director ($X^2 = 6.10$, $2df$, $p = < .047$). By contrast, coordinators in installations with higher status levels tended to prepare and send such reports directly to regional headquarters.

DISCUSSION

Although we are relatively certain that the hypothesis guiding this report was sustained by the data analysis, we are less certain about how to explain our findings. There seem to be at least six possible explanations, which we advanced earlier in this paper. We have either to choose from among them or to speculate on how they can operate in combination in order to explain the differential adoption and use of an alcoholism policy by status level within our sample work organizations. We incline toward the latter approach, but believe we should first examine each dimension singly in order to interpret further how they might act together. For this purpose, we can divide the six into two major categories: those forces causing lower-status drinkers themselves to be more visible in the work place, and those forces causing supervisors to tend to use the alcoholism policy more vigorously with lower-status employees than with higher-status ones.

Prevalence of Problem Drinking

In an effort to counteract the skid-row image of alcoholism that was especially common in the 1950s and 1960s, recent observers have tended to emphasize the number of problem drinkers in middle and upper social classes (Mulford 1964). In the process, the impression has been conveyed that problem-drinking employees are rather evenly distributed throughout the status structure, both in the broader community and in specific work places. Actually, there is still no definitive evidence as to whether problem drinking is more prevalent in some social status levels than in others. What has been available is evidence that problem drinkers are *not* heavily concentrated among the very bottom segments of American society, as the skid-row image would lead one to believe, but are also to be found in sizeable numbers in all other strata. For example, a summary bulletin published by the New York State School of Industrial and Labor Relations at Cornell University in 1959 that brought together practically all extant data (Trice 1959) showed that although problem drinking was not uniquely concentrated in the lower-status occupations, the proportions of alcoholic workers in the clerical, semiskilled, and unskilled categories nonetheless outnumbered high-status alcoholic employees (executives, owners, and professionals) by almost two to one (roughly 40 percent and 20 percent, respectively, of the total number of alcoholic workers). Straus and Bacon's earlier data (1951), which were included in that summary, had shown much the same trend. So did a report on the occupational backgrounds of hospitalized alcoholics almost a decade and a half later, with some exceptions (Ethridge and Ralston 1967).

Despite these forerunners' reports, observers of the industrial scene have found it difficult to accept the later findings of Cahalan and his associates (Cahalan et al. 1969; Cahalan 1970; Cahalan and Room 1974) that show problem drinkers to be three times more prevalent in the lowest than in the upper middle and highest social classes. Compared with the earlier data, their findings were based on a more comprehensive and inclusive definition of problem drinking (i.e., drinking troubles or high-consequence drinking); the studies of the 1950s had used a narrower definition that focused on alcoholism as a more advanced health problem. Also, the Cahalan data differed in that they were obtained from national probability samples of people living in households, and thus presumably included respondents who did not work.

Furthermore, our experiences in work-world research suggested that lower-status people tend to talk more freely and honestly than higher-status employees about their drinking behavior. In fact, our detection of such differential response patterns forced us to abandon usage of Mulford's scale (1964) for measuring the quantity and frequency of alcohol consumption. Perhaps the same kind of reactivity was operating when Cahalan's interviewers came to a household. For that matter, the relative openness and forthrightness of supervisors of lower-level employees in our present study may have led to differential reporting of usage of the alcoholism policy that did not match actual usage. That is, there may well be a class-linked willingness among lower-status persons to divulge drinking patterns more fully than will members of higher status groups. In support of this argument, Trice found that lower-status alcoholics who were members of Alcoholics Anonymous "frequently described their participation [in off-the-job drinking groups] as relatively uninhibited. Thus, they often got drunk with persons from the job with few reservations. Higher-status alcoholics, however, participated in such activities but were very careful to drink 'normally' waiting until they had separated from work associates to drink heavily while alone" (Trice 1962, p 17).

Despite the questions just raised, the combined force of the data in the studies cited suggests that we should reexamine the commonly held belief that problem-drinking employees are distributed more or less equally across occupational statuses. The issues raised should perhaps best be considered as possible moderators of the Cahalan and other data indicating large differentials in drinking patterns according to status. The general pattern may be true, but the size of the differences may have been somewhat exaggerated in the most recent data by some of the factors mentioned. Suffice it to say that one reason for the relatively heavier use of the alcoholism policy at the lower skill levels at the federal installations studied here may simply be that there are more problem drinkers there—making them more obvious, and policy use more relevant for a supervisor of those employees.

Certainly, data show some other forms of deviant behavior to be more prevalent in the lower than in the middle classes, just as there are some forms of deviance that are more prevalent in the middle class than in the lower. For example, psychiatric symptoms among nonhospitalized populations seem more common among the lower classes, as shown in the classic "Stirling County" study, where occupational level was taken to be roughly indicative of socioeconomic position (Leighton 1963). An equally well-known study of noninstitutionalized persons of the same period was the Midtown Manhattan Project—a study in a heavily urbanized area, as the Stirling County study had been completely rural. Langner and Michael (1963) reported that the mental health risk of the lowest socioeconomic group in Manhattan was found to be greater than that for the middle and upper strata there. Yet the stresses that the lower group encountered, as defined by the researchers, were not much greater than those encountered by people at higher status levels. Apparently, persons in the lower socioeconomic groups tend to display psychiatric symptoms in reaction to stress more than do persons at higher status levels. There is abundant evidence that schizophrenia is heavily concentrated in the lowest strata of community life (Roman and Trice 1967; Kohn 1974), where occupational roles are not only of low status, but are also highly unstable. Much the same general pattern was discerned at somewhat higher status levels in Kornhauser's study of occupational status and mental health (1965). The "outstanding finding" of this study of automobile workers was that "mental health varies consistently with the level of jobs the men held; when we compare the factory workers by occupational categories, the higher the occupation" with respect to skill and associated attributes of variety, responsibility, and pay, "the better the average mental health. This finding is even more striking since it occurs within the limited range represented by the comparatively secure, well-paid auto workers of this study" (Kornhauser 1965, p. 262).

Again, going outside the status structure of the work organization to that of the larger community provides a parallel. Both anomie and alienation progressively increase as occupational status decreases (Mizruchi 1960; Rushing 1971), suggesting that an overall value orientation or mode of adaptation emerges from the differential strains and burdens experienced largely by those lower in the social structure (Merton 1949). In sum, there are good reasons to assume both that there is a higher prevalence of alcoholism among lower-status employees and that this higher prevalence reflects a more generalized class-linked tendency toward related deviant behaviors and the value orientations that are consistent with them.

Covering Up and the Visibility of Problem Drinking

In and of itself, a higher percentage of problem drinkers in lower-status jobs means merely that supervisors *may* be more affected by them. It does not necessarily mean that they are therefore actually visible as such and thus require supervisory action. Existing data, however, clearly suggest that this is indeed the case: lower-status problem drinkers and their work performance tend to be much more visible to supervisors and fellow workers than those in higher-status jobs. An earlier report (Trice 1962) demonstrated that within two separate studies of the job behavior of AA members, those in low-status positions were uniquely visible in their work efficiency, absenteeism, cover-up patterns, and on-the-job accidents. Those members who worked in service, semiskilled, and unskilled jobs described themselves as "periodics," whose work was impaired by absenteeism and sharp declines in work performance before and after absences, while higher-status workers tended to come to work persistently, go through various motions, but do practically nothing while there. In short, the work performance of the latter group was just as impaired as the former, but the impairments of higher-status workers were far less apparent to their co-workers. As summarized earlier, "The decline in efficiency of lower status problem drinkers appears to center around visible absenteeism and the period before and after absences. In contrast, alcoholics on more responsible jobs expressed their job inefficiency by a steady mediocre performance, intermingled with occasional absences and spurts of unusual performance'' (Trice 1962, p. 502). Consequently, respondents in the higher-status jobs had much less of the kind of absences that are made more visible by their unreported nature and their back-to-back duration. Higher-status deviant drinkers tended to show up at work no matter what shape they were in, producing more easily concealed ''on-the-job'' absenteeism—at least, more easily concealed in the short run. Failure to appear would spotlight the executive, whereas physical presence acts to deny deviant behavior and thus slows down its detection.

In addition, upper-status jobs often contain more latitude for performance variations, giving their holders an opportunity to catch up later. Thus, their job impairment can be and often is more cyclical than that of their lower-status counterparts, giving them opportunities to recoup. By contrast, many lower-level jobs require physical alertness that can be obviously affected by hangover and/or on-the-job drinking. In past research high-status alcoholics reported significantly more ''self-cover-up,'' while lower-status alcoholics described cover-up experiences provided largely by work associates or no cover-up experience at all while at work. The total lack of cover-up experiences was especially prevalent with low degrees of job freedom—i.e., in cases where a worker had very little, if any, right to decide his own work pattern and pace or to come and go as he wished. Low cover-up was related to low ''freedom from supervision''—a second measure of overall job freedom. Adding further to these workers' risk of detection was their higher exposure to on-the-job accidents, with all the potential for intense investigation that such accidents hold. High-status executives and professionals enjoyed substantial protection from potentially revealing accidents due to faulty machinery, moving vehicles, falling materials, and other hazards (Trice 1962).

Results also indicate that alcoholism among lower-status persons is generally more visible. A study of samples of just over 400 patients from the Toronto Clinic of Alcoholism and Drug Addiction Research Foundation reported by Schmidt et al. (1970) found alcohol excess among lower-class patients to be generally more extreme and to lead to various alcoholic complications more rapidly than among higher-class patients. Consequently, in the lower-class patients ''specific alcoholic symptoms and alcoholic psychoses and acute alcoholic episodes requiring hospitalization are comparatively frequent'' (Schmidt et al. 1970, p. 93). Further, Schmidt and his associates found that the regular use of alcohol among high-status patients seemed less likely to result in overt signs of extreme intoxication.

Intense field observations of four alcoholic presidents (three of well-known companies and one of an international union) agree with these findings and further illuminate how high-status alcoholics receive thorough cover-up and protection at work—in sharp contrast to low-status AA members, who often reported no cover-up experiences at all (Trice and Belasco 1970). A small clique of lieutenants both covered up for and exploited these high-level executives for their own gain. Consequently, the presidents appeared to many subordinates to be going about their executive duties in a regular manner and drinking the way other executives do. The clique members closely supervised morning drinking, on-the-job drinking, and heavy afterhours drinking; the executives were carefully escorted starting in mid-afternoon to make certain that deviant drinking was well camouflaged. In effect, these presidents traded off a large measure of their power and authority for the protection they received from their trusted lieutenants. In so doing, they typify the "successful" deviants (Roman 1974) who are able to use resources at their disposal from their middle- and upper-status levels to avoid "getting caught." They are, in effect, like a large majority of respectable middle-class people who have committed felonies but have not been caught.

Moreover, the very status of these middle- and upper-strata "successful deviants" implies that they have invested heavily in conformity through hard work, diligence, and prudent behavior. Consequently, they view themselves as having more right to deviate, more right to be tolerated, protected, and covered up than do lower-class workers, who are, they believe, deviants from the American values of achievement, success, cleanliness, and material possessions. Additionally, high-status employees, because of formal education and numerous opportunities for wider experiences in organizational life, are probably more clever in their deviations than their lower-class counterparts. They better understand how to exchange clique relations, how to maneuver the subtleties of power, and how to control sources of information.

Higher-status drinkers also are often aided in their self cover-up by their greater opportunities for privacy, which in turn provide opportunities to engage in deviant drinking without being detected. Lower-status employees control far less space, and their deviant drinking will more readily disrupt the on-going job pursuits of others, bringing on negative social sanctions. When opportunities to avoid detection are joined by freedom to set work hours—job features typically enjoyed only by high status personnel (Trice 1962)—they produce a set of forces that operate to produce low visibility on the job; conversely, high visibility occurs where such features are not operating.

Social Distance as a Component in Differential Policy Use

The higher prevalence and higher visibility of problem drinkers in low-status jobs clearly puts greater pressure on their supervisors to use the alcoholism policy, making it substantially more salient for them. These two forces, however, do not necessarily overcome the reluctance of supervisors to exercise available sanctions. Theory and research findings suggest that it is easier for persons to exercise social controls over those who are seen as "different" from them (Goffman 1963). It seems obvious that our supervisors, by virtue of being in a managerial job, were in some sense differentiated from their subordinates, regardless of their skill level. It is also likely that this social distance (or the degree of perceived difference) may have been more pronounced for supervisors of low-status employees, especially those supervisors who had advanced through several of the promotion steps of the federal civil service, which was the case for many supervisors in our sample, since it was representative of all hierarchical levels. In other instances, supervisors may be hired on different bases than lower-status employees; supervisory status may, for example, require a college degree, while subordinates lack college training. But those supervisors at the professional skill levels, defined as involving a college degree or the equivalent, may not differ in their education and occupational status from their subordinates. And supervisors who also belong to a profession may derive their primary social status from the occupation, rather than from their position in the managerial hierarchy, which is of secondary importance in status terms.

Thus we conclude that part of the reason that the alcoholism policy was used differentially on low-status problem drinkers was because there was sufficient social distance between them and their supervisors to produce a willingness to use social sanctions (the policy) against them. Problem drinkers at higher skill levels with less routine jobs may be perceived by supervisors to be more similar to themselves; the lessened social distance between them and their subordinates may cause them to be less universalistic in applying formal policies to those subordinates. Perceived similarity tends to reduce social distance, encourage informal social relations between supervisors and supervised, and thus encourage particularistic orientations. Moreover, high-skill-level employees are probably in a more advantageous position to generate "power equalization" vis-à-vis their supervisors (Emerson 1962; Beyer 1975). That is, they can engage in behaviors that reduce the power exercized over them by their supervisors, either through more effective coalition formation or through their greater opportunities to cultivate alternative employment. Finally, at high skill levels, supervisor and supervised often share a common occupational commitment and identity, such as that found among accountants, lawyers, or social workers, including value orientations and other commitments that further serve to reduce social distance between them.

What evidence is there that such explanations fit the data reported here? Numerous findings uphold such an interpretation. For example, as reported above, supervisors of a mixture of skilled and professional employees, or of professionals only, were much more likely to manage alcohol-related absenteeism by keeping it between themselves and the employee, a clear violation of the policy (universalism) and an equally clear indication of informal management between supervisor and supervised (particularism). This finding represents a refinement of a major finding in an earlier study concerning the organizational and attitudinal forces playing on supervisors to both discourage and encourage them to use an alcoholism policy (Trice 1965*b*). The chief discouraging factor was a strong sentiment among most supervisors to handle the matter themselves rather than use company policy and procedures. It seems quite likely, in the light of these current findings, that a large proportion of the supervisors holding these sentiments were supervisors of higher-status employees.

Our data also showed that supervisors of lower-skilled subordinates were much more likely to issue an official reprimand or take other disciplinary action—universalistic acts that suggest substantial social distance between supervised and supervisor. A similar argument can be made for the comparative tendency of supervisors of the less skilled to use discharge more often and never resort to transfer, which was a substantially frequent action by supervisors at higher skill levels. On the other hand, Warkov and associates (1965) report that supervisors, once they identified employees as problem drinkers, more frequently assigned negative ratings to those at skilled and white-collar levels, a finding they interpreted to mean less tolerance of deviant drinking at middle status levels and greater tolerance for that at lower status levels.

Interestingly, a large-scale, tightly controlled evaluation of supervisors' training on problem-drinking employees found that supervisors showed substantially more willingness to confront and take a universalistic approach to a problem-drinking employee following a training intervention that created social distance between themselves and such employees (Trice and Belasco 1968). These findings support the hypothesis that supervisors often hold a rather favorable view of the problem drinker rather than a stigmatic one. Until this is reversed, creating a sense of social distance, of perceived difference, between supervisor and subordinate, the supervisor will be reluctant to apply the policy. Apparently this sense of difference was significantly stronger among supervisors of low-status employees in our current study, helping them to make use of a policy that applied to a personnel problem that was also relatively more salient for them.

Risks and Punishments Associated with Applying the Policy

Supervisors of highly skilled employees probably face substantially more risks, perhaps even sanctions, in applying the alcoholism policy. If this is true, it further explains the findings. Unfortunately, no systematic data exist for this interpretation. We do have, however, rather careful notes of spontaneous responses that did not fit directly into the format of our instruments. That is, field interviewers prepared special data forms to record these unanticipated responses, and supervisory comment on them, in as much detail as possible. Repeatedly, supervisors of highly-skilled and professional employees voiced deep concern about the risks they ran in using the alcoholism policy. These risks were: (1) giving their unit a bad name; (2) having known problem drinkers in highly sensitive and responsible jobs when their performance, they believed, had been permanently damaged; (3) having somehow to substitute for problem drinkers even though they had received treatment and even though the supervisor did not have personnel with whom to replace them; and (4) having to disrupt their budgets because of the high cost to them and the functioning of their units of such employees being in treatment, combined with the high cost to the unit of finding replacements when the returned and treated alcoholic professional could not be trusted in a highly sensitive assignment. In general, they felt that the policy as presently worded did not take into sufficient account their unique situation as supervisors of high-priced, highly trained, talented employees in occupational situations where they had not expected any alcoholics to begin with and where continued problem drinking was considered intolerable because of the associated risks mentioned above. Some observations in this vein suggested they would "work with what we've got" before running the risks they saw in the policy requirements and recommendations. They saw few organizational rewards for themselves in using the policy and voluntarily indicated, far more often than supervisors of lower-status employees, that they saw the policy as punishing to themselves. Apparently such supervisors believed that the high-status alcoholic would "snap out of it" sufficiently, could be transferred sooner or later, or would respond to retirement opportunities to avoid policy use. Furthermore, the policy was too formal; if some informal means could be found to do what the present formal policy attempted to do, they would probably be more receptive—comments supporting our social-distance explanation.

The volunteered comments of lower-skill-level supervisors contained none of these concerns. They spoke rather freely of the likelihood of misconduct in general among their employees, appearing to be sensitized to its presence. Their comments had a tougher, "hard-hat," first-sergeant flavor, suggesting that they saw no risks in policy use and even saw opportunities in it to prove that they could do a good job: "Most of my men have only a grade-school education, and you have to bring them into line when they hit the bottle too much," or "You have to prove to them [subordinates] that you won't take any drinking crap from them—and you can't play favorites for such guys.'' Numerous unsolicited comments from these supervisors suggested that they saw the policy as helping them control their subordinates and as providing them with an opportunity to continue to demonstrate their toughness ''upstairs.'' In a sense, they seemed to imply that they needed to use McGregor's Theory X as a supervisory style—an approach that emphasizes a rather pessimistic view of employee potential and motivation combined with a belief in ''going by the book'' and conforming with the formal bureaucracy and its policies (McGregor 1960). Furthermore, instead of seeing risks in using the policy, those who volunteered additional comments suggested that the policy would help them with problem employees in general and alcoholics in particular: ''You have to keep a close eye on him because he's a safety hazard, and the alcohol thing backs me up if I have to take action next time he is out—and he is out a lot.'' Another supervisor of low level employees commented: ''He was a bad influence on the other men and on me too—I never knew what to expect next—so this policy came along when I really needed it.'' And another: ''He was putting me in a bad light, and I needed to do something about him, and I did something—with the help of my boss I used the booze policy.'' Although these observations are only proffered remarks generated by formal research instruments, they suggest an unexplored dimension of policy use, namely organizational rewards and punishments that supervisors perceive accruing to them if they activate the policy.

A Combined Explanation

Apparently, the higher prevalence and visibility of problem drinkers at the lower-status job levels makes for policy salience among supervisors of such employees. At the same time, these managers probably experience more social distance between themselves and their subordinates, facilitating policy use. This relative readiness to use the policy among supervisors of low-status employees is further reinforced by few perceived risks in its use and by relatively more rewards.

IMPLICATIONS

The findings and interpretation presented above suggest that differential means for implementing alcoholism policies, according to the overall skill level of a work organization on the one hand and the various skill levels within it on the other, should be considered. For example, it seems obvious that high-status supervisors perceive the policy quite differently and use it much less. Differential attention should be given to them even though they probably experience less alcoholism among subordinates. For supervisors of higher skill levels, written forms with an emphasis on impaired work performance, which they appreciate, seem to work best to generate increased familiarity with the policy. Union familiarity with a policy is more helpful at this level in producing use of the policy, and if no union is present, then rank-and-file familiarity has roughly a similar effect. Coordinators should be appointed as early as possible and given training, especially in the use of community resources and in understanding the risks higher-status supervisors believe they face in applying the policy. Also they probably need more staff help. Finally, since the tendency of high-level supervisors to handle the drinking problems of their personnel on a private, personal basis badly impedes implementation, special attention should be given to this barrier. Training which will create feelings of social distance between these supervisors and their subordinates is clearly indicated. An emphasis on general supervision, as compared with specialized, occupational know-how, is clearly suggested. Within such a framework, alcoholism could be better dealt with in such a way as to avoid "backlash," keeping in mind that drinking problems may understandably be less salient for the higher status levels, for all of the reasons already mentioned.

For supervision of lower skill levels and low-status employees, implementation could be tailored around an emphasis on oral forms of policy communications that also underscore impaired job performance, but in a fashion that recognizes that this central policy feature is not currently understood by these managers. In addition, supervisors at this level need to be urged, in some fashion, to understand the constructive, helping thrust of the policy, so that they do not overuse its disciplinary features with their subordinates. Their clear desire for additional information about the policy should provide an opportunity for training programs that spotlight positive policy provisions. Coordinators are probably much more effective with these supervisors if their official appointment is widely emphasized and if they are provided with tools for further increasing the feelings of supervisors that the policy can assist them in the management of a difficult personnel problem.

Much the same general conclusions seem to apply to community treatment resources. High-status alcoholics referred to them will tend to come from, and return to, very different occupational circumstances than do low-status alcoholics. In all likelihood, adaptations of therapeutic techniques to this basic fact would be appropriate. Practically nothing is known about such adaptations, but these findings strongly suggest that they badly need to be explored. For example,

Mayer and Myerson (1970) report that improvement in work performance occurred in just over 40 percent of the high-status employees who underwent outpatient therapy, while only 4 percent of the low-status employees showed such improvement. Apparently, the higher use of the policy on lower-status employees found in this research may not be compatible with outpatient treatment; perhaps this is one reason disciplinary actions were used so frequently for this group of employees.

REFERENCES

Bendix, R., and S. M. Lipset, eds. 1966. *Class, Status, and Power*. New York: The Free Press.

Beyer, J. M. 1975. "Power dependencies and the distribution of influence in universities." Unpublished paper, School of Management, State University of New York at Buffalo, 25 October 1975.

Cahalan, D. 1970. *Problem Drinkers: A National Survey*. San Francisco: Jossey-Bass.

Cahalan, D., I. H. Cisin, and H. M. Crossley. 1969. *American Drinking Practices: A National Study of Drinking Behavior and Attitudes*. New Brunswick, N.J.: Rutgers Center for Alcohol Studies.

Cahalan, D., and R. Room. 1974. *Problem Drinking among American Men*. New Brunswick, N.J.: Rutgers Center of Alcohol Studies.

Emerson, R. M. 1962. "Power-dependence relations." *American Sociological Review* 27:31–41.

Ethridge, D. A., and J. A. Ralston. 1967. "Occupational backgrounds of institutionalized alcoholics: Comparative data and implications for rehabilitation." *Mental Hygiene* 51:543–48.

Goffman, E. 1963. *Stigma*. Englewood Cliffs, N.J.: Prentice Hall.

Kohn, M. 1974. "Social class and schizophrenia: A critical review and a reformulation." In H. M. Trice and P. M. Roman, eds., *Explorations in Psychiatric Sociology*. Philadelphia: F. A. Davis.

Kornhauser, A. W. 1965. *Mental Health of the Industrial Worker: A Detroit Study*. New York: Wiley.

Langner, T., and S. Michael. 1963. *Life and Stress and Mental Health*. New York: The Free Press.

Leighton, D. 1963. *The Character of Danger*. New York: Basic Books.

McGregor, D. 1960. *The Human Side of Enterprise*. New York: McGraw-Hill.

Mayer, J., and D. J. Myerson. 1970. "Characteristics of out-patient alcoholics in relation to change in drinking, work, and mental status during treatment." *Quarterly Journal of Studies on Alcohol* 31:889–97.

Merton, R. 1949. "Social structure and anomie." In *Social Theory and Social Structure*. Glencoe: The Free Press.

Mizruchi, E. 1960. "Social structure and anomie in a small city." *American Sociological Review* 25:645–54.

Mulford, H. 1964. "Drinking and deviant drinking, U.S.A." *Quarterly Journal of Studies on Alcohol* 25:634–50.

Roman, P. 1974. "Settings for successful deviance: Drinking and deviant drinking among middle- and upper-level employees." In C. D. Bryant, ed., *Deviant Behavior: Occupational and Organizational Bases*. Chicago: Rand McNally.

Roman, P., and H. M. Trice. 1967. *Schizophrenia and the Poor*. Ithaca: New York State School of Industrial and Labor Relations, Cornell University.

Rushing, W. A. 1971. "Class, culture, and 'social structure and anomies.'" *American Journal of Sociology* 76:857–62.

Schmidt, W., R. G. Smart, and M. K. Moss. 1970. *Social Class and the Treatment of Alcoholism*. Toronto: University of Toronto Press.

Straus, R., and S. D. Bacon. 1951. "Alcoholism and social stability: A study of occupational integration of 2,023 male clinic patients." *Quarterly Journal of Studies on Alcohol* 12:231–60.

Trice, H. M. 1959. *The Problem Drinker on the Job*. Bulletin 40. Ithaca: New York State School of Industrial and Labor Relations, Cornell University.

———. 1962. "The job behavior of problem drinkers." In D. J. Pittman and C. R. Snyder, eds., *Society Culture and Drinking Patterns*, pp. 493–510. New York: Wiley.

———. 1965*a*. "Alcoholic employees: A comparison of psychotic, neurotic, and 'normal' personnel." *Journal of Occupational Medicine* 7:94–99.

———. 1965*b*. "Reaction of supervisors to emotionally disturbed employees." *Journal of Occupational Medicine* 7:177–88.

———. 1966. "The alcoholic employee and his supervisor." In R. E. Popham, ed., *Alcohol and Alcoholism: Papers Presented at the International Symposium in Memory of E. M. Jellinek*, pp. 338–46. Toronto: University of Toronto Press.

Trice, H. M., and J. A. Belasco. 1968. "Supervisory training about alcoholics and other problem employees." *Quarterly Journal of Studies on Alcohol* 29:382–98.

———. 1970. "The aging collegian: Drinking pathologies among executive and professional alumni." In George Maddox, ed., *The Domesticated Drug: Drinking among Collegians*, pp. 218–34. New Haven: College and University Press.

Trice, H. M., P. M. Roman, and J. A. Belasco. 1969. "Selection for treatment: A predictive evaluation of an alcoholism regimen." *International Journal of the Addictions* 4:303–17.

Tumin, M. M. 1967. *Social Stratification: Form and Functions of Inequality*. Englewood Cliffs, N.J.: Prentice-Hall.

Warkov, S., S. Bacon, and A. C. Hawkins. 1965. "Social correlates of industrial problem drinking." *Quarterly Journal of Studies on Alcohol* 26:58–71.

FOUR / Unionism and Alcoholism: The Issues

LEO PERLIS

Many union members are producers and sellers as well as consumers of alcoholic beverages. They work in distilleries, breweries, vineyards, package stores, and bars. That is how they make their living. Many more union members are part of a vast army of drinking Americans, and some of them, for one reason or another, have lost control and surrendered to the habit—always totally and often irrevocably. That is how they lose their living and, sometimes, even their lives. It should not be too difficult, therefore, to understand labor's early ambivalence about movements designed to prevent and control the manufacture and sale of alcoholic beverages. It is somewhat similar to labor's current ambivalence about cigarette smoking.

THE EVOLUTION OF LABOR'S POSITION ON ALCOHOLISM

In the early 1950s when the National Congress of Industrial Organization (CIO) Community Services Committee established a formal relationship with the National Council on Alcoholism, the president of the Brewery Workers complained. His concern was full employment for his members, and he feared that crusades against alcoholism could quite easily be converted into crusades against alcohol. This reasonable fear of forced idleness was coupled with the working man's tendency, in an earlier day, to identify whiskey drinking and beer guzzling with manhood and fun. Drinking a companion under the table was a boast not entirely lost, even in these less macho days. Unlike many other Americans, union men and women on the whole never took to the axe like Carrie Nation nor to the streets like the Women's Christian Temperance Union. Neither were they great fans of Congressman Volstead. Indeed, it is entirely possible that during Prohibition, some union men spent a considerable amount of time ringing bells in the less exclusive speakeasys, stomping grapes in their home-made wine cellars, or crying over a mug of near beer in the corner saloon. As late as the mid-1960s, a high official in the American Federation of Labor and Congress of Industrial Organizations (AFL-CIO) proposed, only half-jokingly, to the director of the

AFL-CIO Department of Community Services that he "lay off this alcoholism bit," adding quite seriously: "Don't be a party pooper."

In addition to these inherent contradictions in the American—and perhaps even in the universal—social and economic order, organized labor faced still another problem: management attitudes. Drinking on the job was often tolerated in an open shop but frequently punished during organizing drives. Union men suspected that the boss took it out, not so much on the drinking employee, as on the demanding employee: their often well-founded suspicion was that alcoholic intoxication became a euphemism for union agitation. Whether or not these suspicions were always justified, they remain, albeit to a lesser degree, to this very day. It is no wonder, then, that union men and women covered up for the alcoholic. If the "ruthless" company boss was intent on firing him, the "faithful" union friend was just as determined to defend him. It has taken many years of developing union security and management enlightment to bring about the kind of acceptable labor-management relationships which have in recent years resulted in joint labor-management concern for the alcoholic. This changed attitude is perhaps best symbolized by the establishment of the Labor-Management Committee within the National Council on Alcoholism, under the cochairmanship of George Meany, president of the AFL-CIO, and James M. Roche, former board chairman of the General Motors Corporation.

How does labor look upon the alcoholic now, in this age of public confession? In different ways, of course—traditional, conventional, and up-to-date. There was a time when a drunk was a drunk, and if you didn't lecture him, pity him, lock him up, or save his soul, you simply laughed with or at him. But you didn't think of him as a person with a disease, either physiological or psychological. To help the drunk you might have called the preacher but hardly the doctor. Labor shared these attitudes (and guilt feelings) along with other Americans. In the jungle of the unknown and unproved, workingmen accept the conventional wisdom of the day. As laymen, they have no alternative. And so it was that when the disease concept of alcoholism was accepted widely by a number of professional organizations, such as the World Health Organization, the American Medical Association, and the U.S. Public Health Service, labor refused to speculate and simply went along. In 1958, in an article entitled "Do Insurance Companies Cover Alcoholism as a Disease?" based upon a study of 50 insurance companies, the director of the AFL-CIO Department of Community Services raised the question, "Is alcoholism a disease?... Has acceptance [of alcoholism as a disease] been converted into practical coverage by the health insurance companies of the United States?" And he answered his own question: "The movement to gain recognition for the disease concept of alcoholism will have been finally won only when it is fully covered by health insurance companies."

Labor's acceptance of alcoholism as a disease does not go beyond current conventional wisdom; it extends neither to the mystique of the arrested alcoholic nor to the fashionable dogmas of the day. It is a commonsense approach. Since nobody knows precisely the causes and cures of alcoholism, it makes sense that the alcoholic must stop drinking—while research and experimentation continue in behavior modification, chemotherapy, and other modes of treatment.

The patient, then, is of first concern. Union programs today are neither pro-union nor pro-management but pro-patient. While management is often concerned with the alcoholic first as a productive worker and only second as a human being, labor looks upon the alcoholic first as a fellow worker with a problem. Absenteeism, turnover, productivity, and production are all secondary. Labor believes that the end product of sound emotional health is not increased productivity but sound emotional health. Increased productivity is only a practical by-product. This difference in emphasis is often at the heart of labor-management misunderstandings and disagreements in the development and promotion of joint programs for the prevention, treatment, and recovery of alcoholics in industry. As more cooperative relationships are established, however, controversy may be greatly reduced, if not entirely eliminated.

GOALS OF TREATMENT AND REHABILITATION

The AFL-CIO, which represents some 14.5 million organized workers associated in 110 national and international unions and more than 60,000 locals, has stressed from the very beginning that such cooperative relationships can be established only through the development of proper organizational machinery. In organized plants, this machinery would include the following:

—Union-management committees on alcoholism.
—Jointly agreed guidelines on methodology.
—The training of union and management representatives from top to bottom on jointly agreed policies, programs, and procedures.
—Provision for keeping alcoholism outside the arena of controversial negotiations wherever possible.
—The inclusion of procedures for handling alcoholism in the collective bargaining agreement.

—Provision of insurance coverage for alcoholism as a disease.
—The protection of job security and seniority.
—The establishment of counseling and referral procedures.
—Respect for established grievance and arbitration procedures under the union contract.
—Concentration on alcoholism without resorting to such euphemisms as "broad brush," "troubled employee," or "employee assistance."
—The involvement of both labor and management in community-wide efforts to establish adequate facilities for the treatment and recovery of alcoholics.

By and large, union members no longer shy away from calling an alcoholic an alcoholic. This forthright approach, most labor leaders feel, is the first step to recovery. The inability of an alcoholic to recognize and to admit his alcoholism should be understood but not approved. The most successful recovery program to date, Alcoholics Anonymous (AA), is based on direct self-confrontation, self-examination, self-confession, and self-control. In the absence of something better, this approach is widely accepted in the labor movement. Calling an alcoholic worker "a troubled employee" is like calling an alcoholic physician "a troubled professional." Neither does much except divert our attention from the target: the alcoholic.

But what if the alcoholic employee is unable to recognize his disease and refuses treatment? What if all union, management, and professional efforts fail? Should the alcoholic worker (or for that matter the alcoholic executive) be fired? The answer to this question is another question: What is the alternative? Obviously there is none. Unions recognize that an alcoholic who refuses treatment is not only on the road to ultimate self-destruction but is an unfair burden to his employer, his fellow workers, his family, and the community as a whole. In the last analysis, firing the unrepentant drunk (to use an old-fashioned, moralistic phrase) after everything else has failed, from early soft-soaping to final hard-lining, may be therapeutic for everyone—including the alcoholic himself. To avoid unfair action, controversy, and recrimination, the discharge of an employee, even for good and sufficient reasons, should be handled strictly in accordance with the spirit and the letter of the collective bargaining agreement.

Most union officials, possibly as a result of their relatively low economic background, activist training, and bargaining experience, are direct. They dislike circumlocution, and they distrust indirection. Nor do they like job bugging and medical snooping. Problem identification and referral "based entirely on deteriorating job performance criteria" may be sold by some eager-beaver personnel people and professionals to a few unsuspecting labor officials, but most trade unionists do not buy this approach. In the first place, incipient alcoholics do not always perform poorly. In the second place, even hardened drunkards have been known to perform well for a time. In the third place, it is important to reach all problem drinkers, including those who work well, instead of waiting until their job performance deteriorates. Finally, problem drinkers may not be the only ones to perform poorly. There are also problem gamblers, problem consumers, problem husbands and wives, problem neighbors and fellow workers, and problem people generally. To convert what should be a purely alcoholism detection, referral, and treatment program into a "broad-brush troubled-employee assistance program" covering every personal, social, economic, and behavioral problem is not only diversionary and unscientific but pie-in-the-sky to boot. That, of course, isn't to say that alcoholics don't create other problems for themselves as well as for their families and that something shouldn't be done about it. It is to say, however, that the best way to deal with workers' personal and family problems in organized plants is for unions and managements to establish joint programs and procedures on a broader "health and welfare" basis, dealing forthrightly with all health and welfare problems through collective bargaining, counseling and referral procedures, insurance coverage, and other systems.

As for the alcoholic and the problem drinker, more and more unions in recent years have joined with corporate executives to devise programs based on the following five *r*'s: (1) recognition of the alcoholic as a sick person; (2) respect for the problem drinker as a fellow human being; (3) referral of the alcoholic to appropriate professionals and agencies for treatment; (4) restoration of the alcoholic to useful citizenship and productive employment; and (5) readjustment of the alcoholic to the battle of life and work, without resorting to the bottle.

Is the battle for life and in the work place more difficult for unorganized employees than for unionized workers? Do union men and women drink less than their counterparts in unorganized plants? Do certain occupations cause more tensions (and, therefore, more drinking) than other occupations? Do union men and women stop off at the bar for a drink or two before going home more or less than nonunion men and women? In short, is union membership and security, per se, helpful in the prevention of problem drinking? While there are no comparative studies into the extent of alcoholism among organized and unorganized workers, the labor movement is aware that the disease respects neither industrial nor jurisdictional lines.

Still, perhaps something can be learned from research into occupational and trade union influences in the making of an alcoholic. In the absence of conclusive scientific evidence pointing to either psychological or physiological factors as the prime causes of problem drinking, occupational tension and union security cannot be ruled out entirely as important factors in the cause or prevention of alcoholism. But whatever the cause and whatever the cure, unionism and alcoholism are now bound together by virtue of the fact that union members can be—and often are—alcoholics too.

PART II

FIVE / Kennecott's INSIGHT Program

OTTO JONES

On 1 July 1970, the Utah Copper Division of Kennecott Copper Corporation developed a program for its employees and dependents having any kind of problem. Literally a pretreatment-intervention method, it is often referred to as a "troubled people" or "broad-brush" program. INSIGHT, a program of help by referral, provides an easy way people in need to secure professional assistance through the proper community resources.

FEATURES OF THE PROGRAM

INSIGHT offers not only a service, but confidentiality, self-determination, and convenience. It accepts referrals from all sources, ranging from the Employee Relations Department, unions, and supervisors, to friends, family, and relatives. It has eliminated all red tape; one need only dial the letters I–N–S–I–G–H–T (467–4448) and a 24-hour-a-day, seven-day-a-week counseling service is at his or her disposal. Anyone may contact INSIGHT and report a problem affecting an employee. The program will guarantee anonymity for the caller and the person referred. If the person accepts INSIGHT's offer, help is given; if not, the counselors politely back away.

The mechanics begin with a call to INSIGHT. The caller is then referred to the program director, a psychiatric social worker, for counseling. Problems are discussed and alternative solutions utilizing community resources are made available. The employee or relative then makes a decision and a referral is made. Follow-up is very important to make sure the referred individual received the necessary help. Sometimes another referral is required.

Employees who begin to develop chronic absenteeism or poor job performance patterns are offered help before the problem gets out of hand. To accomplish this goal, assistance is offered in the areas of alcoholism, drug abuse, family problems, marital problems, indebtedness, legal problems, etc. Whatever the reason, referral to INSIGHT permits getting to the root cause and in many cases solves the problem and saves the employee's job.

INSIGHT is built into the company disciplinary procedure, on the premise that the sooner an employee with a job-performance or absenteeism problem gets help, the better his chance for keeping his job will be. Normally, an employee who is performing unsatisfactorily or absent excessively will first be given a verbal warning. If improvements are not made, a written warning follows. Continued misconduct warrants a hearing with the employee, his union representative, and the Employee Relations Department. Probationary terms are usually issued at this point. The next and final step in the disciplinary procedure is termination.

With each of the above contacts with the employee, INSIGHT is also notified. INSIGHT's approach then is to offer assistance: the employee's involvement in the program is never mandatory. In each instance a sincere attempt is made to help the troubled employee, and in the vast majority of cases, the services are gratefully received and appropriate corrections made. Employee morale is greatly boosted when employees realize that the company will take an interest in problems and offer help rather than issue an insensitive, mandatory stipulation of "compliance or else." Loyalty toward the company and the job is the prevailing result.

To make maximum penetration possible, information regarding the program and its potential must be effectively disseminated. This is accomplished through direct letters to the employees, special bulletins, company magazines, television spots, and presentation through lecture to the front-line supervisors and union personnel. Explanation of program mechanics lowers anxiety and speculation regarding involvement. The best means of advertising, however, is through positive feedback from those having had experience with INSIGHT.

COMMUNITY ORGANIZATION

It is the responsibility of INSIGHT to maintain a working rapport with community social service agencies and all other facilities that might be made available to Kennecott employees and their dependents for whatever problems they might have. To accomplish this, INSIGHT must not only acquaint itself with community resources, but become a part of community planning. There are some interesting public relations dynamics involved here. Every year the Utah Copper Division receives many requests for community project donations. Often in the past, these contributions remained just that—contributions. Today, the company considers these contributions more in terms of an investment, beneficial both to Kennecott Copper Corporation employees and to the community at large.

INSIGHT has a follow-up procedure through which the participating persons indicate to the staff just how adequately they are being helped. This enables the program to give valuable feedback information to the community social service agencies and private facilities to whom Kennecott people have been referred. INSIGHT, therefore, becomes active in upgrading existing resources and in making recommendations for improvement. Indeed, one of the most exciting aspects of the program has been its impact on the health care delivery system. Through pretreatment preparation for referral, an arrangement is made for follow-up on the person(s) involved. The professional and the patient both recognize the need to move in and out of treatment as quickly as possible. Even those professionals who tend to be susceptible to unethical practices realize the scrutiny and, because they do not wish to be confronted, quite often police themselves. The more effective, efficient practice that is encouraged is manifest through reduced hospital, medical, and surgical costs. Peer group committees and utilization boards can also contribute to more economical health care delivery. The patient, too, can play a part by keeping a log of services rendered to be compared with a copy of the paid claim from the insurance company. Whenever a discrepancy is discovered, it is reported to the INSIGHT office for further investigation.

THE GOAL OF EARLY IDENTIFICATION

It seems paradoxical that when dealing with a progressive illness such as alcoholism, an assistance program should dictate that problems should be manifest in job performance before intervention is justified. This is as ludicrous as telling a person who has cancer (after the recognition of the disease in the prodromal phase) to go out and get a little worse and come back for treatment when the problem is chronic. I say this because the profile of the inebriate detected on the job is a person over 45 years of age who has been working for a particular company for 15 to 20 years and has been drinking for at least that long. Obviously, this describes an individual rapidly approaching the chronic phase of alcoholism. Therefore, our emphasis is on secondary prevention efforts. Primary prevention is education seeking to prevent a person's leaving the social drinking category and going over into the continuum of alcoholism. Secondary prevention can be applied during that period of time between the initial phases of alcoholism and the chronic phases. Although INSIGHT might not be able to prevent a person from having a problem with alcohol, it might be in a position to intervene before the problem becomes chronic.

This pretreatment-intervention method that concentrates on secondary prevention is the most effective approach in terms of penetration into the problem of alcoholism known today. One reason is that through the encouragement of voluntarism, a family might seek help, presenting a problem that is not the primary problem at all. For example, a man may present a marital problem, complaining that he and his wife do not communicate well any more. His wife agrees but has an additional complaint about his drinking. Thus, the marital problem presented becomes potentially secondary to a possible primary problem of alcoholism. Of course, such accusations require further investigation and scrutiny before final determinations are made. Therefore, a professional staff qualified in differential diagnoses is necessary, since the INSIGHT program deals with all problems, not just alcoholism.

The concentration on secondary prevention is also effective because the program not only makes referrals to the community but organizes the community to make referrals to it. The courts are a good example of this system. It is recognized that incarceration is not much of a deterrent to anything, especially in the case of the public inebriate, as recidivism makes clear. The judicial system readily cooperates with therapeutic alternatives to these punitive measures. Thus, arrangements are made for the court to make referrals as an alternative to fines and/or incarceration. Of course, the individual is still not coerced into utilizing the "troubled people" program. INSIGHT does, however, use the leverage of the court for those who are willing to keep the individual involved in treatment. And, if the individual reneges on the agreement to stay involved in therapy, through follow-up, the courts are notified, and his original obligation can be met through normal judicial means. Very often, INSIGHT is given the opportunity to work with an employee having a drinking problem before it becomes manifest on the job.

Financial companies are also encouraged to make referrals to INSIGHT on any employee who might be a candidate for a garnishment. Financial problems occur for reasons, and often they are related to alcohol problems. This, then, enables INSIGHT to offer assistance to the problem drinker during the earlier phases of the illness.

School districts are also contacted. Whenever a child of a Kennecott employee is having a problem within the educational system, the district is asked to refer the child to INSIGHT. The counselors, in turn, contact the family and acquaint them with INSIGHT and the ways in which it might be of assistance to them. INSIGHT has never, as yet, been rejected. The usual response is one of relief and encouragement. Quite often it is found that families have exhausted their alternatives for solving the problem and are glad to have someone intervene with new possibilities for consideration. It is not uncommon to discover that marital difficulties with underlying alcohol problems are causing the disruption that is affecting the child's school performance. Before a treatment plan is designed for the child, he or she is given a physical and psychological examination. Speculation is thereby reduced, and a more appropriate approach to the problem can be made.

EVALUATION

The need for an accurate, up-to-date system of records is self-explanatory. It provides INSIGHT with a reliable means for measuring current response and for evaluation. It assists in making program adjustments and documents history. Closely related to the rationale for records is the need for accurate research. Currently, INSIGHT is trying to upgrade its own services and effectiveness in an attempt not only to accommodate but to encourage program participation. To date, our research has included a preliminary study for program justification and comparison. This was followed by a study within the plants to check absenteeism and job performance improvements of those employees who were referred via the disciplinary procedure.

The most recent study was completed midway through the program's thirty-second month, in February 1973. A sample of 150 men who had used the INSIGHT program was observed on a before-and-after basis. We calculated their absenteeism, weekly indemnity costs; and hospital, medical, and surgical costs over a six-month period before their involvement with INSIGHT, compared with a six-month period immediately following their program involvement. After an average of 12.7 months in INSIGHT, these 150 men improved their attendance by 52 percent, decreased their weekly indemnity costs by 74.6 percent, and decreased their hospital, medical, and surgical costs by 55.4 percent.

INSIGHT services produce positive results in relation to alcoholism and other personal and social problems. It is apparent that absenteeism can be reduced considerably by providing people with social services for problem solving. This is accomplished by continuous, up-to-date knowledge of community resources, shared with the individual according to need and interest. Such a program improves morale, enhances employee relations, and better integrates industry into the community's activities. Benefits are realized by both the individual and the company. Periodically INSIGHT informs the employees of the program's progress and utilization. This not only supplies them with information about the program's current activities but also serves to keep them aware that the program continues to operate. Without such information, impetus falters and enthusiasm dwindles.

CONCLUSION

Some challenge the right of business and industry to intervene in the personal lives of employees and/or dependents, feeling that this "big-brother" notion is threatening to confidentiality. But one must challenge their accusations by questioning their right to speak on behalf of potential program participants. The program is not for people who do not need it but for those who do, and it is the experience of INSIGHT that many people have been very pleased to have this service available when they needed it. Voluntarism is encouraged, and the users of the service are made aware that they are in no way obligated. The service is free of charge, and no one is coerced into following any of the recommendations or counsel of the staff. It is important that the name of the program does not identify with any particular problem, for to do so creates a stigma and inhibits utilization, especially in the case of alcoholism and/or drug abuse.

Although referrals are received through the disciplinary system, it has been the experience of the Kennecott INSIGHT Program that only 15 percent of its case load comes through this method. This seems to be congruent with the penetration rate of all industrial programs that concentrate on the disciplinary system as their only means of referral. We have found that reaching out, following up, maintaining a simple system to encourage utilization, and implementing a monitoring device that establishes quality control are all elements conducive to success.

SIX / The Program for Alcoholism at Metropolitan Life

WILLIAM R. CUNNICK, JR., and
EDGAR P. MARCHESINI

Metropolitan Life has traditionally been concerned about problems that adversely affect the welfare of its policyholders and employees. As far back as 1909, when our Health and Welfare Division was organized, we established positive action programs to campaign against tuberculosis and other infectious diseases. We were also concerned about maternal and child health, sanitation, and other major health problems of the times. Later, we expanded our public educational programs to include diabetes, heart disease, cancer, mental health, accident prevention, alcoholism, and drug abuse. The reason for our concern is simple: people are our business. Whatever helps people live longer, healthier lives concerns us.

HISTORY OF THE PROGRAM

In 1919, we established the position of housemother in our home office in New York City to help employees with problems related to their business life or to some purely personal, nonmedical matter. This informal counseling service continued through 1943. In 1949, anxious to reestablish this service for the benefit of the home office clerical staff, which then numbered 13,000, the company's president appointed Dr. Lydia Giberson to the post of personal advisor. Dr. Giberson, with 17 years of company service in the Medical Division, had developed an excellent reputation for helping home-office people with nonmedical problems. In undertaking this new assignment, Dr. Giberson discontinued her connection with the Medical Division and was given independent status as a member of the president's staff. During her tenure as personal advisor in the home office (1949–61), she expanded employee counseling to include medical and behavioral problems. Simultaneously, in the 1940s and 1950s, an unpublicized alcoholism program to conserve the health and valuable skills of employees with serious drinking problems was developed in the home office and in the field under the guidance of the medical director and the personnel officer.

In 1951, Metropolitan published a booklet entitled *The Alcoholic* which was made available to the public. At that time, alcoholism was considered to be a moral rather than a health problem. It was common to characterize alcoholics as people who were dissolute, weak-willed, and dangerous. Popular magazines with nationwide distribution printed the booklet's message about the dangers of alcoholism, and we received numerous compliments from readers for bringing this controverisal problem out into the open. Requests for the booklet exceeded those for all other titles offered during 1951 in such widely read magazines as the *Saturday Evening Post, Time,* and *Good Housekeeping*. Ultimately, 500,000 copies were printed and distributed to readers throughout the United States and Canada. In 1960, we followed up with a new booklet addressed to the public, *Alcoholism: A Guide for the Family,* which was also received most favorably. It described various treatment modalities and attempted to erase the age-old stigma associated with this insidious health problem.

During the period 1951–60, the informal alcoholism program developed by the Medical and Personnel Departments took root. It resulted in the formation of the Chairman of the Board's Committee on Alcoholism, comprised of officers of the Medical Department and other home office departments. In 1960 this committee formulated a written policy on alcoholism that was distributed initially to officers and division managers in the home office and, later on, was introduced into our field operations. The written policy was introduced to company officers at a monthly officers' luncheon in the home office in 1960, at which time the implementing procedures and the role of the supervisor were also explained. Subsequently, Medical and Personnel Department specialists met with supervisors and managers throughout the home office at regular monthly staff meetings to distribute copies of the policy and to explain their role in carrying out the new policy and program.

From its beginning, the Alcoholism Committee had strong support from top management. In fact, the Alcoholism Committee, later renamed the Alcoholism and Special Problems Committee, continued to function as a policymaking body until 1973, when it was replaced by a Medical-Personnel organizational arrangement. (At that time, a large– scale company reorganization required streamlining of all committee activities.)

Shortly after the introduction of the alcoholism program in the home office, Dr. Giberson retired, and her counseling function was incorporated into a new unit within the Personnel Department called Employee Advisory Services. This unit, established in late 1962, was headed by a knowledgeable personnel specialist, Eugene Hill, who had worked closely with the Medical Department over the years in counseling employees with drinking problems. Staffed by highly qualified laymen who had demonstrated exceptional skills in working with employee problems, the new counseling unit was designed to broaden the base of employee counseling. In addition to providing confidential counseling on personal and job-related problems, the staff was equipped to advise employees on retirement planning, money management, and budgeting. It worked in tandem with the Medical Department in administering the company's alcoholism and drug rehabilitation programs.

POLICY AND OBJECTIVES

Employee Advisory Services conducts more than 3,500 interviews annually with employees in the home office and in regional and district sales offices. The unit handles about 85 percent of the cases referred to it and has access to other company departments and community resources when specialized help is needed. From the inception of the alcoholism program, we have gone to great lengths to assure confidentiality of information relating to any employee participating in the program. The careful protection of the employee's anonymity has paid big dividends in the form of increasing self-referrals, which might otherwise have been unobtainable.

The company's policy on alcoholism reads as follows: "Alcoholism or excessive drinking is a serious health problem leading to progressive mental and physical deterioration. When an employee's drinking adversely affects work performance, it becomes a matter of company concern." The policy statement indicates that "no employee should be denied help in the treatment of this disorder." It also stipulates that no disciplinary action will be taken against an employee who cooperates in rehabilitation, makes progress, and maintains a satisfactory performance record.

Under the implementing procedures, the supervisor is asked to make referrals either to the Medical Department or to Employee Advisory Services strictly on the basis of work performance and to avoid any subjective evaluations or judgments as to the nature of the problem causing the unsatisfactory job performance observed. The diagnosis of alcoholism as well as the selection of appropriate therapy is clearly defined as a function of the Medical Department.

The supervisor's role in dealing with behavioral problems involved the following steps:

—Verify that the employee's performance is deteriorating as evidenced by precise documentation.

—Limit criticism to overall job performance and avoid trying to diagnose the employee's underlying problem.
—Document examples of poor job performance or excessive absence and lateness. Be specific and factual regarding the date, time, place, and nature of the incidents.
—Discuss all aspects of the problem with his or her immediate superior.
—Arrange for a confidential interview with the employee, discuss the poor work performance, and make it clear that if work performance does not improve, disciplinary action will have to be taken.
—Suggest that the employee visit the Medical Department or Employee Advisory Services to discuss whatever problem is adversely affecting job performance.
—If job performance continues to deteriorate because the employee refuses all offers of help, denies a problem, or does not cooperate or respond to treatment, then appropriate disciplinary action should be taken. This may include discontinuance of active employment.

The confrontation interview is a technique we find useful in breaking down the "denial defense" of employees with alcohol-related problems. Besides the employee, the participants in this crucial meeting are the medical director, the divisional officer or manager, the Employee Advisory Services representative, and, if possible, the employee's family. The value of the organized confrontation interview is that it prevents the problem employee from playing off one party against the other. In addition, it assures that all aspects of the alcohol-related problem will be given proper attention. This is very important because alcoholism is a total disorder that adversely affects all facets of the problem drinker's life. Employee Advisory Services' main role in the rehabilitative process is to monitor the employee's progress and to help the alcoholic resolve any secondary problems that may have negative repercussions on work performance and rehabilitation. Some of the problems created by excessive drinking have marital, familial, financial, and legal implications, and, if unresolved, can lead to recidivism.

One of our earliest problems following the establishment of the alcoholism program was in communicating the policy to all levels of employees, especially supervisory and managerial personnel. We resolved this problem by printing appropriate articles in our bimonthly magazine and weekly newspaper. Later, the program was briefly described in the *Employees' Handbook* and in the *Personnel Policies and Procedures Manual,* as well as through various training programs for new employees, first-line supervisors, and managerial personnel. Members of the Medical Department and Employee Advisory Services participate in these educational activities, which are designed to stimulate group discussion.

One of our most serious concerns is the failure to identify the problem drinker during the early stages of the disease. What is called early detection in industry is too often identification of the employee in the middle or late stages of alcoholism, after serious job problems have already developed and at a time when the prospects for successful rehabilitation may be lessened. We have been trying to overcome this obstacle by impressing upon management the need for prompt action at the earliest signs of an underlying problem evidenced by job deterioration, attitudinal changes, and patterns of excessive absenteeism and lateness. Our Medical Department has been effective in detecting alcoholics who have not yet developed poor work habits through periodic health examination. An integral part of the periodic examination includes the SMA 12 blood test. Metropolitan purchased an SMA 12/30 AutoAnalyzer in March 1967 and used it to obtain biochemical profiles on 1,000 employees on whom we had detailed medical information. The purpose of the research was to determine whether the new equipment would enable us to diagnose organic conditions in their incipient stages. One of the unexpected by-products of this test was that it indicated possible alcoholic liver disease in otherwise apparently healthy persons by abnormal readings of SGOT (serum glutamicoxalacetic transaminase), an enzyme which when present in the bloodstream in elevated amounts indicates the destruction of liver tissue. The Medical Department has found that employees with drinking problems who are confronted with these biochemical profiles are often willing to admit to a drinking problem and accept help. Although this method is not foolproof, it certainly has enhanced our chances of detecting the early-stage alcoholic.

Diagnosing alcoholism at a beginning stage has presented some problems in treatment. Earlier-stage alcoholics have more difficulty in understanding the seriousness of the illness and are less ready to accept the Alcoholics Anonymous (AA) message with its goal of sobriety. They complain about the horror stories, the sameness of the meeting format, their inability to identify with AA members, or their feeling that the AA approach is too evangelistic. Some feel that they can overcome alcoholism through controlled drinking programs that promise to curb alcoholism and convert them into social drinkers. In our opinion, these individuals have more drinking to do and are not ready for any kind of help. Although we as a company wholeheartedly endorse AA and feel that it is the most successful program for helping alcoholics achieve sobriety and, more importantly, peace of mind, in the few special cases that are not receptive to AA, the Medical Department and Employee Advisory Services staff follow up more closely to get a better understanding of their therapeutic needs. If the underlying problem seems to have an emotional basis, the employee may be referred to a psychiatrist or to group therapy. In some situations we utilize in-house recovered alcoholics in a one-on-one relationship or any combination of resources that may achieve positive results. In other words, we use an eclectic approach with regard to individual rehabilitation. We think it is important to keep an open mind about new approaches to treatment and to recognize that rehabilitation of the alcoholic employee is a long, tortuous, and even frustrating experience. However, it is certainly worth our best efforts when it results in recovery.

During the past several years Metropolitan has been involved in an extensive reorganization. We have been establishing a regional organization throughout the United States to reduce costs and improve services to our policyholders. As these dispersed offices are established across the country, we are faced with the problem of setting up viable alcoholism programs at each one. Although the organizational problems are not insurmountable, it is difficult to implement and administer a company policy and program in a multibranch operation. Not only is there a geographical problem, but there is also the added responsibility of establishing procedures that will assure uniformity in policy application. The problem is further compounded because the employees in dispersed offices, especially newly appointed management personnel, have not had sufficient time to familiarize themselves with corporate policies and philosophy. Initially, management in these recently created offices is primarily concerned with recruiting, selecting, and training employees; providing adequate facilities and services to carry out office functions; establishing contact with the community; and the myriad other details related to becoming operational. Under these circumstances, it seems clear that the implementation of an alcoholism policy will have low priority.

Despite these obstacles, we have already advanced through the embryonic stage in most of our dispersed offices and are beginning to establish viable programs. Employee Advisory Services representatives visit head offices and computer centers with the objectives of acquainting employees and management with the company's alcoholism policy and program; educating managers and supervisors regarding the dangers of substance abuse and briefing them on their role in implementing the policy; establishing effective referral and follow-up counseling procedures; and identifying and evaluating local treatment facilities. Concurrently, the medical director assigns knowledgeable Medical Department personnel to head offices to direct the medical aspects of the program locally. At this stage, they report all cases involving alcoholism to the Medical Department at the home office for review and guidance. Ultimately, the intention is to have them function independently.

Among the problems in setting up a decentralized organization is the monumental task of identifying local treatment facilities and other supportive services. Presently the Medical Department and Employee Advisory Services are working together to identify and evaluate inpatient rehabilitation facilities across the country, especially in areas where we have large concentrations of employees (head offices and computer centers) or group policyholders. We start these on-site inspections by contacting state occupational program consultants, affiliates of the National Council on Alcoholism, AA intergroup offices, etc., for recommendations. Although we intend to investigate all types of treatment modalities in this long-term project, we are concentrating primarily on nonhospital inpatient rehabilitation facilities. In general, these treatment centers direct alcoholic counseling modalities through affiliation with Alcoholics Anonymous, and they provide treatment of longer duration and have less medical identity than do hospitals. In addition, they deal directly with alcoholism, per se, rather than with the treatment of a physical disorder secondary to alcoholism. They are usually less expensive than hospitals providing detoxification and limited after-care, and frequently can achieve more beneficial results.

We have already evaluated some of the better-known primary rehabilitation facilities, such as Hazelden in Center City, Minnesota; Chit Chat Foundation in Wernersville, Pennsylvania; and Smithers Alcoholism Treatment Center in New York City; and we are presently planning visits to similar treatment centers in selected areas. We have developed the following criteria for evaluating inpatient rehabilitation centers:

—Treatment of approximately four weeks' duration.
—Physician in attendance, or at least on call, and nursing service available when necessary.
—Mandatory daily therapy sessions—individual and group—with professional and nonprofessional staff. Disciplines represented would include medicine, psychology, social service, and AA.
—Formal educational sessions—lectures, films, and question-and-answer periods.
—Interviews with spouse and family.
—Chaplain services for various faiths.
—Qualified and experienced counseling staff, with a combination of formal training and experience in helping alcoholics.

—Regularly scheduled AA meetings for patients, with provision for referral to local chapters after release.
—Patient entry centered on those already employed or employable rather than on the street alcoholic.
—Certification by an authoritative governmental or medical body. The facilities should be open for inspection by accredited agencies and business organizations which might wish to refer employees.

The treatment facilities that meet the above standards are usually accepted for coverage under our company comprehensive medical expense plan. In addition to those we have already approved on an individual basis, we are recommending that the company approve for coverage 64 treatment facilities accredited by the Joint Commission on Accreditation of Hospitals as of the end of May 1975.

CONCLUSION

Since we issued the written policy on alcoholism in 1960, the company program has helped many employees at all levels to arrest this insidious problem. Al-

TABLE 6.1 METROPOLITAN LIFE ALCOHOLISM PROGRAM STATISTICAL REPORT, 1961–1972

Cases Recovered or Controlled for Two Years or Longer	
Still in active employment	84
Deceased after two years' improvement	9
Normal retirement after two years' improvement	38
Disability benefits after two years' improvement	8
Resigned from company	8
Total	147
Cases Not Considered Recovered	
Discontinued	57
Deceased	21
Retired under program	2
Disability within two years	7
Total	87

Recovery rate: $\frac{147}{234} = 62.8\%$

Discontinuance rate: $\frac{57}{234} = 24.3\%$

though we have no definite cost figures, we know that the program has resulted in substantial savings to the company. The latest alcoholism program statistical report (see Table 6.1) indicates a recovery rate of 62.8 percent based on a study of 234 cases for the period 1961–72. Our criterion for determining this rate is two years of continued active employment, with improvement in work performance, attendance, and attitude following identification.

We feel that close follow-up after identification is most important to provide needed support and encouragement to the recovering alcoholic. Both the Medical Department and Employee Advisory Services play a major role in the follow-up process. The two years after identification is the danger period, the time when relapse is most likely to occur. If an occasional slip does occur during this critical period, however, it does not necessarily mean that recovery has failed. Prompt action by the Medical Department and the counseling service can help get the employee back on track and even reinforce his or her determination to achieve sobriety.

In the final analysis, we feel that the real value of our alcoholism program is the contribution it makes in conserving the health of employees and restoring them to a useful and productive life. There is no way to measure this value in terms of dollars and cents. The founders of the company alcoholism program were clearly more concerned about human-life values than monetary savings.

SEVEN / Evaluating the New York City Police Department Counseling Unit

REV. MSGR. JOSEPH A. DUNNE

While writing on bureaucracy, Max Weber describes the characteristics of a large police department (Gerth and Mills 1946, pp. 96–198). The commissioner or director heads subordinate commanders having fixed jurisdictional areas of the city. In military fashion, these areas are subdivided into divisions and precincts. Police duty is outlined in minute detail in official publications issued to each member. Strict discipline is exerted to assure the protection of citizens' life and property. Officers with the needed qualifications are selected through civil service procedures and are given special training for a six-month period before receiving a gun and a shield with authority to perform police duty. Policing a city around the clock requires long tours of duty, traditional loyalty, personal responsibility, and a cohesiveness among members seldom seen in any other type of organization. Characteristically, the police officer is "the conscience of the community," enforcing the law for all citizens in all parts of the city, and funneling arrests into the courts for trial and prosecution.

Not surprisingly, therefore, police administrators are frequently puzzled by officers who drink too much. Generally they have not been able or even willing to look at the problem of alcoholism in their ranks from a behavioral and management point of view. I hope to demonstrate in this chapter that police officers suffering from alcoholism can be successfully treated and retained as skilled and useful employees.

DEVELOPMENT OF THE NEW YORK CITY POLICE COUNSELING UNIT

When I was appointed police chaplain in 1958, I learned that my duties required not only visiting the sick, injured, and dying, and administering to the spiritual welfare of the members of the department, but also supervising men placed on probation for disciplinary violations. The charges against these men revealed that the majority had drinking problems that resulted in misconduct, excessive sick time, accidents, and marital difficulties.

I contacted Alcoholics Anonymous (AA), attended the meetings regularly, and sought the assistance of recovered members of the department. I examined the alcoholism programs of the New York City Transit Authority and the Chicago Police Department. I also attended the Summer School of Alcohol Studies at Rutgers University. The knowledge which I acquired firmed up my determination to establish a program for the New York City Police Department.

Overcoming Organizational Resistance

Since I had the assimilated rank of inspector, I was in a position to propose that the department begin to look at the problem-drinking officer with respect to sickness and accident rates, the disruptive effects on disciplinary procedures, the public image of the department, and the possibility of lawsuits against the city when a police officer fired his weapon without authorization. However, most organizations resist any attempts by a "renewal stimulator" to upset the equilibrium of the organization (Lippitt 1969, p. 114). Indeed, the classical reaction of a bureaucratic structure to the proposal of a program to assist alcoholic employees could be easily forecast, given both informal and formal structures of a police organization.

The influence of the informal structure has been aptly demonstrated by Westley (1951). Despite defensive attitudes, Westley succeeded in interviewing a number of police officers in a city near Chicago. He found among them the tightest kind of group cohesiveness—men working closely together against crime and not trusting outsiders. At the same time, these men demanded the highest respect from the public. Thus, under the guise of organizational loyalty, policemen could be expected to "take care of" men who drank heavily before going on duty as well as those who became drunk on duty and as a result got into fights, shootings, and losing gun or shield.

At the formal level, the resistance I found on the part of the chief surgeon when I sought cooperation in initiating a counseling program closely paralleled Dalton's description of the line-staff problems of a factory situation (1959). Moreover, the chief surgeon's lack of empathy for alcoholic officers was communicated to the subordinate district surgeons, who, while they may have wished to assist alcoholic employees, refrained from doing because of the attitude of their superior. Then, too, departmental regulations forbade men on sick report to leave their homes for AA meetings. When a police officer was diagnosed as intoxicated by a surgeon, he was immediately suspended from duty, his guns were removed, and the medical report would indicate that he was depressed, incoherent, or manifesting underlying personality disorders. This harsh treatment resulted in many police officers being transferred to limited duty status, doing clerical work without firearms, with little hope that they would ever be restored to full duty. Fines for intoxication were excessively high and almost automatic. An officer would lose 30 days' pay and then be placed on probation for one year. In view of these punitive measures, superior officers were reluctant to report alcoholics, and this resulted in continued organizational cover-up.

The retirement of the chief surgeon in 1961 gave new hope for the proposed program. Yet the rigidity of the bureaucracy continued, especially on the part of those in charge of public relations, who feared that a counseling unit would impair the image of the department. On 10 February 1962, at my request, a line-staff conference was held with deputy commissioners, chaplains, police surgeons, the chief inspector, and headquarters officers. The deputy commissioner for trials reported that in the previous 11 years, 121 men were suspended for intoxication, with an average of 31.8 days' suspension. The new chief surgeon assured the conference that a majority of the district surgeons favored the idea of instituting a rehabilitation program. The chief inspector, however, spoke of adverse public criticism which might be directed against the department. As a consequence, the recommendations growing out of this conference were not made known to the police commissioner.

Finally, I became convinced of the necessity of obtaining a clear-cut policy at the top level of mangement. Together with people in the Personnel Department, I submitted a memorandum to the police commissioner outlining the plans for a counseling service. The chief surgeon also wrote an official request recommending that a counseling unit with AA therapy and a hospitalization program be formed, promising the active participation of the district surgeons. This coordinated effort outlined the current enlightened view of alcoholism in industry, generated official reports of the past performance of the department in assisting problem drinkers on an informal basis, and expressed the concern of the surgeon and the chaplain that the medical and welfare problem be met honestly. This memorandum was delayed in channels for another year.

On 12 May 1966 Commissioner Howard Leary, after discussing the proposed program with the surgeon and the chaplain, signed a departmental policy on alcoholism. A brief summary of this policy is as follows:

—Alcoholism is a disease and the alcoholic a sick person requiring skilled rehabilitative assistance.

—Alcoholism is a departmental health problem and therefore a departmental responsibility.
—Each officer with suspected alcoholism or problem drinking shall be encouraged to seek adequate medical advice and counseling without delay.
—Support and assistance will be afforded to any employee who cooperates and displays a sincere effort at rehabilitation.
—Records will be kept strictly confidential.
—Problem drinking will be considered to exist for the individual when his duty performance is materially reduced in efficiency and dependability because of drinking when such drinking is not an isolated experience but is more or less repetitive and when such drinking results in recognizable interference with health or personal relations.
—Each commanding officer will be responsible for the early detection of problem drinking on the part of any member of his command and for prompt referral for rehabilitative assistance.
—The department's primary purpose is to rehabilitate the alcoholic to the status of a sober, reliable, productive employee, thus retaining his skills, training and experience. In cases where all available rehabilitation attempts have failed, termination of employment on a consistent and equitable basis is in the best interest of the department.

Informal and Formal Phases of the Unit

Until May 1966, the Counseling Unit operated on an informal basis; and the chaplain, with the help of police members of AA, received referrals from family members, disciplinary trials, the Medical Unit, and a few supervisors. Police officers did not relish recording complaints against fellow officers, especially from family members who risked violent reaction at home. As a consequence, these complaints were frequently ignored at the precinct level. Job conflicts, on the other hand, are departmental problems. The supervisor cannot tolerate deterioration in the quality of work, and he must deal with the active alcoholic. Fellow members grow tired of covering his mistakes, and the problem drinker often then goes through a personality change. His friends do not enjoy his company or his prolonged drinking; they resent his hostility, and he becomes a loner. He now drinks to relieve tention, resentment, and loneliness; and in so doing actually perpetuates the addiction. Indeed, in a study of 36 employed male alcoholics referred to the New York University Consultation Clinic for alcoholism, Hurwitz and Lelos (1968, p. 70) reported that 70 percent were in conflict over their dependency wishes.

In its informal stage, the Counseling Unit conducted interviews with 73 persons (of whom 32 were hospitalized); 34 of these cases were referred by the Medical Unit. In contrast, during the first 13 months of the unit's formal stage, a total of 216 persons were interviewed, and of these, 163 were referrals from the Medical Unit; 104 admitted having a problem, and 79 were hospitalized. This influx was attributed to better case finding in the Medical Unit, whereby a large number of suspected problem drinkers were uncovered from medical records, specifically from the chronically sick list.

Because of the hazards of police service, the department has a policy of unlimited sick leave granted by the city of New York. The department must monitor those employees who call in sick. A person is considered chronically ill if he is out for this reason more than six times per year. Thus, examination of the medical folders of the chronically sick uncovered numerous instances of Monday morning sickness that were termed gastroenteritis or stomach disorder, which often signifies coming off a drunk. Personnel officers also made a regular survey of accident records, paying particular attention to bizarre activities, especially those instances where an officer lost a gun or shield; where a gun was discharged; or where the lateness of the hour implied that the employee was out drinking. When a police officer was suspected of or arrested in connection with intoxication, on or off duty, he was contacted by a member of the Counseling Unit and interviewed for the purpose of hospitalization and rehabilitation. The sick member frequently saw a possibility of early restoration of duty if he cooperated with the department's counseling service. A comparison of the first year's activity during the formal stage with that during the informal stage shows that the department's formal program had a greater degree of penetration into the organizational problems of alcoholism.

THE TREATMENT PROGRAM

The work flow of the Counseling Unit, an in-house treatment program, is outlined in Figure 7.1. The treatment program begins with the referral, the source of which may be the Medical Unit, family complaints, a chaplain, or the Employee Relations Unit. Referral leads to case findings and then to the initial interview.

Initial Interview and Medical Determination

The combined efforts of trained supervisors, counselors, and medical referrals of suspected problem drinkers reaches its first test of effectiveness in the initial

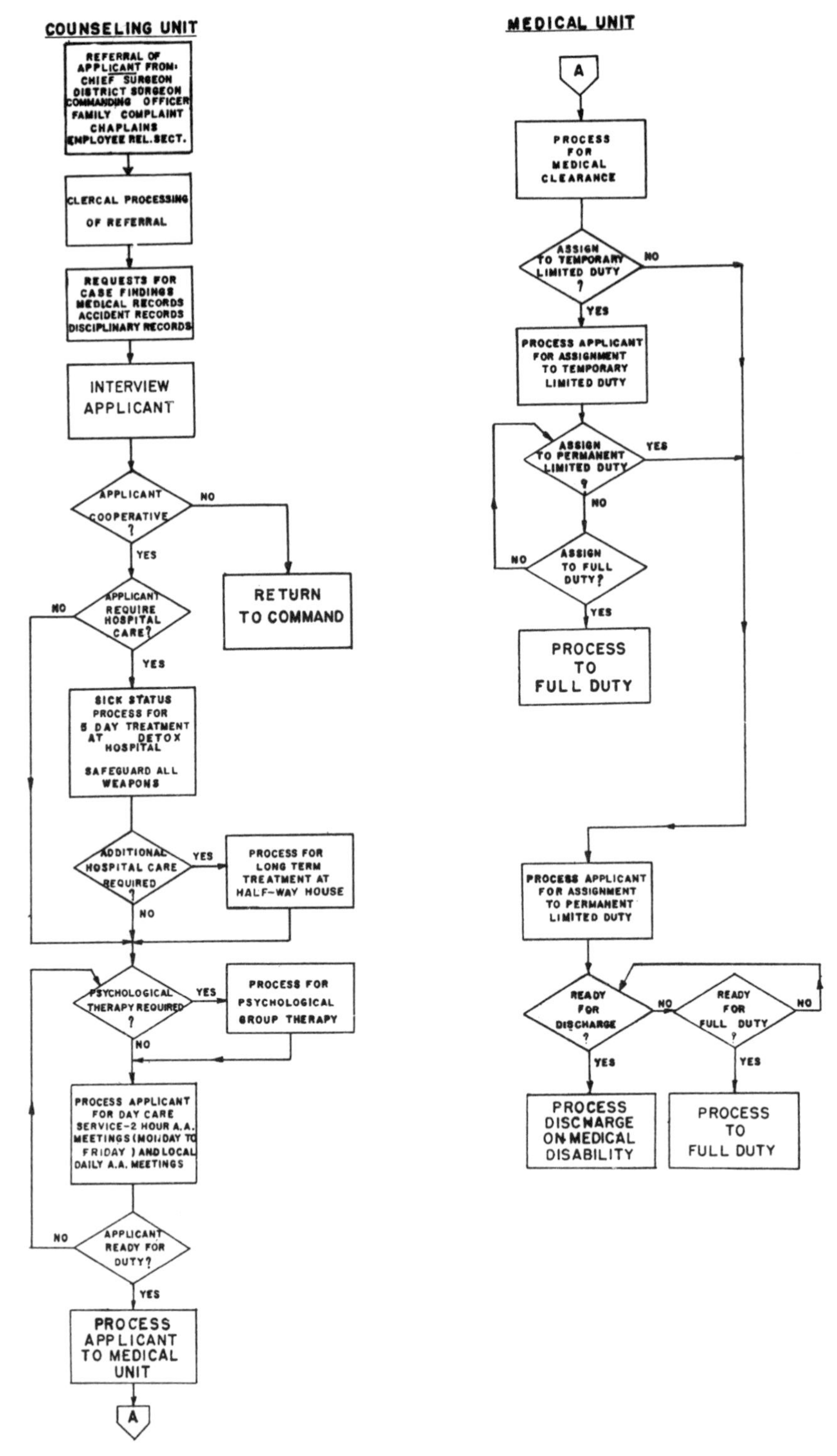

FIGURE 7.1. NYCPD Counseling Unit: Work-Flow Chart.

interview. The counselor is a police officer in civilian dress who is a recovered alcoholic. All his talents and experience are brought to play as he greets his fellow officer, who has been ordered to report for this interview.

Most problem drinkers are fearful of endangering their job, highly sensitive to the term *alcoholic,* and very resentful about being required to discuss their private affairs. Even officers suspended for intoxication are often convinced that they have been given "a bad break." The approach taken in handling the alcoholic employee must therefore be a delicate one. As C. E. Wilcox states (1968, p. 78) the counselor must realize that this interview is likely to be unpleasant; he should expect to be confronted with denials, excuses, rage, remorse, lies, and promises. Dr. Harry M. Tiebout (1965, p. 496) writes that the alcoholic is absorbed in his grandiosity and defiant individuality until he reaches a point of desperation. Dr. Tiebout calls the process of getting the alcoholic to cooperate and accept treatment "inducing therapeutic surrender."

After attempting to put the employee at ease and assuring him that the records of his drinking experience will be kept confidential, in accordance with departmental policy, the counselor begins to record the progress of the illness on a chart adapted from that used in the Consolidated Edison Program (see Figure 7.2). A profile of advancing alcoholism is drawn on an age basis, beginning with social drinking and moving through the problem drinking to the chronic stages. Various symptoms, identified by Dr. Jellinek (1946), are noted by the counselor, and a line is drawn down the chart, illustrating to the employee his life story in terms of alcohol. Thus confronted with the evidence that he himself has submitted, the employee may become more aware of the seriousness of his drinking problem. The reverse side of the chart is then utilized to record the patient's accident record, medical history, and disciplinary infractions, as well as the counselor's comments and recommendations for treatment. The counselor follows up with "Twelve Questions," published by Alcoholics Anonymous, in order to determine the amount of insight the employee has into his drinking problem.

The chaplain, as director, reviews the work of the counselor in the presence of the patient. Here, the role of the chaplain is seen as a friendly one, dedicated to the ministry of assisting police officers and their families. He reinforces the findings of the counselor and goes on to discuss the impact of drinking on the officer's family life. He uses his position to advise the employee to cooperate and accept whatever assistance may be offered as beneficial to himself and to his family.

If the patient is still undecided about whether or not he has a drinking problem, he is referred to the Medical Unit for an interview with the chief surgeon or his

MEDICAL UNIT

NAME ______________________ DATE ______________________

SHIELD NUMBER ______________________ COMMAND ______________________

REFERRAL ______________________ AGE ______ DATE APPT'D. ______

PROFILE OF ALCOHOLISM

STAGES

STAGES											
1. SOCIAL DRINKING											
2. DEPENDENT DRINKING											
Excessive drinking											
Relief of tension											
3. PRE-ALCOHOLIC											
Sneaking drinks											
Gulping drinks											
Blackouts											
4. PROBLEM DRINKER (loss of control)..											
Abnormal behavior											
Evening drunk											
Weekend drunks or on days off											
Drinking on job											
5. ALCOHOLIC											
Morning drink											
Water-wagon											
Solitary drinking											
Changing pattern											
Rationalization											
6. CHRONIC ALCOHOLIC.................											
(a) Benders extend into week											
Acute auditory hallucinosis											
Delirium tremors											
First hospitalization											
(b) Almost continuous drinking											
Anxieties											
Sedatives											
Protecting supply											
Alcoholic neurities											
Alcoholic cirrhosis											
7. ORGANIC DETERIORATION											
Chronic brain syndrome											
Alcoholic psychosis											
AGE	20	25	30	35	40	45	50	55	60	65	

DIAGNOSIS: ADDICTIVE DRINKER ☐ HABITUAL EXCESSIVE SYMPTOMATIC DRINKER ☐

STAGE ______________________

FIGURE 7.2. NYCPD Medical Unit: Profile of Alcoholism.

deputy. Here the doctor reviews the medical record, discusses the findings of the counselor with the patient, and urges him to cooperate by joining the department's counseling program. The doctor can send him on to a hospital or, in some cases, refer him to AA meetings in the community. If the patient is completely lacking in insight and cooperation, a decision must be made regarding his welfare, independent of his reaction. If a man is not a chronic alcoholic and is in good physical condition, he may be returned to his unit with an appropriate warning by the doctor to abstain from alcohol. If the uncooperative patient is obviously suffering from an advanced stage of alcoholism, however, both the chaplain and the doctor will use their strongest moral persuasion to get him to accept hospitalization. Here, his job can be used as a lever to get compliance, based on the terms of the department's policy. Frequently, too, a phone call to the employee's wife robs him of his last defense, as she is happy that his problem has been brought to the attention of the Medical Unit and that he will receive assistance.

Detoxification

Speaking of alcoholism treatment, the American Medical Association's *Manual* (1968) says: "Most clinicians agree that hospitalization is indicated in the early phases of most treatment programs, especially if there are apparent or suspected physical complications or when it is clear that intervention is needed to interrupt the drinking pattern." The vast majority of police alcoholics are convinced by the police surgeon that they need hospitalization immediately. In recognition of the danger of sudden withdrawal, a five-day stay at Columbus Hospital in New York City is usually recommended. Here, the patient is placed on a medically supervised plan of withdrawal and on a reduced program of nonaddictive medication. He receives a high intake of vitamins, including B-12, and can be expected to return to normal physical health during his five-day treatment. During the hospitalization period the patient attends lectures on the disease of alcoholism, several AA meetings, and group therapy sessions in order to convince him that he has a problem. Personal identification and admission to himself that his problem is alcohol is considered of paramount importance to this stage of treatment.

After a five-day stay, the patient feels better and has greater self-confidence but is advised that he is not yet fit for work. He is directed to an additional three-week stay at a halfway house far removed from the city. There, he enjoys rest, light physical exercise, and a substantial diet. His knowledge is deepened with a daily schedule of meetings at the house and in the community. His tutor in this AA way of life is a director who has had 21 years of sobriety and is qualified to give personal guidance. Informal discussion groups and learning experiences reveal problems and relationships which lie at the root of guilt, resentment, and tension. Here, the removal of barriers to emotional and intellectual growth can be accomplished. Wasted years of drinking have taken their toll, and a fantasy world has been substituted for reality. The alcoholic finds it hard to face reality in other people and even in himself without the help of his fellow alcoholics (Clinebell 1968, p. 174). The patient's family is often encouraged to visit him over the weekend and to participate in appropriate conferences and social activities at the lodge. Many husband-and-wife relationships have been stabilized and normalized in this helpful setting.

Limited-Duty Assignments and Restoration and/or Retirement

Thus far, the patient has been on sick report under the control of the chief surgeon and the Counseling Unit. Upon his return from the halfway house, he will be seen by a doctor and then placed in a limited-duty assignment. For most individuals, immediate return to active duty is not yet indicated even though they are no longer drinking. The Medical Unit retains administrative control over the patient for 90 days, and this assignment is extended whenever it is deemed necessary for therapeutic reasons. The officer is then assigned to day tours at police headquarters units and will attend a regular two-hour therapy session weekly at the Counseling Unit. He is also required to attend an AA meeting each evening in the community and to report this activity to his therapist. The record of meetings attended together with weekly reports on changes of attitude, appearance, and cooperation are entered into his folder at the Counseling Unit for evaluation when determining return to full duty.

After a period of 90 days or longer, the case is reviewed, and a decision is made as to whether the police officer may return to his former command. The policy is to test his recovery in a realistic manner, with familiar faces and problems, as well as to impress his fellow workers with the effectiveness of the counseling program. If the patient returns to drinking during this period, a new effort must be made on his behalf, possibly including hospitalization, psychological group counseling, and/or psychiatric assistance. Here, however, he may feel the sanction of the organization, for his firearms, which were temporarily safeguarded, may now be permanently removed, and he will be assigned to permanent limited duty in view of his lack of cooperation. If a patient is deemed unable to recover from alcoholism in the opinion of his chief surgeon, or if he has been on limited duty for more than one year, he becomes eligible for retirement for physical disability. Fortunately, alcoholism is considered an ordinary disability in the personnel practices of the City of New York.

IMPACT OF THE COUNSELING PROGRAM

In the past ten years, the experience of the New York City Police Department in counseling problem drinkers indicates that 75 percent can be returned to full duty as police officers. Some of the benefits which accrued to a group of 50 men illustrate what can be done through a counseling program.

A Study of 50 Patients Interviewed by the Counseling Unit, 1967–68

Three years following interview, 84 men were picked in sequence using a table of random digits. Those who had refused treatment, had denied that they had a problem, or had retired, been dismissed, or died during the three years since interview were eliminated, leaving a total of 50 for analysis. The disciplinary and medical records of these 50 patients who completed the therapeutic process were compared before and after treatment (Dunne 1973). Information voluntarily given in the initial interview regarding age, years of service, and the point at which drinking had progressed was used as a basis for this study.

Most of the men had been alcoholics for almost nine years before they were admitted to the Counseling Unit, the majority having become alcoholics between the ages of 21 and 30 (mean age, 28.6), but having been interviewed largely between the ages of 30 and 45 (mean age, 37.4). The average number of years of service which members of this group rendered before coming to the Counseling Unit was 17. This average, combined with the high incidence of disciplinary charges (disciplinary charges had been experienced by 38 of these men), is evidence that the department was slow to take cognizance of problem drinkers in its ranks. These statistics also show that supervisors attempted to cope with the problem on a disciplinary level, failing to recognize it as a medical problem. The mean number of disciplinary charges per man (2.3) was more than twice the rate for the department as a whole. Following treatment, this group of employees returned to duty, and no disciplinary charges were placed against them, a record that could be viewed as a significant contribution of the Counseling Unit to organizational effectiveness.

A significant and useful comparison in this study was the number of sick absences for all reasons before and after treatment. The mean number of days used for sick leave in the 12 months before counseling was 35. Following treatment, for the 12 months after return to duty the average sick time was 16.8 days—a reduction of more than 50 percent. It is also noteworthy that 20 of the men had no sick time whatsoever after returning to duty. Although little information on alcoholism was available in the medical records of the department before 1966, when the Counseling Unit was formally established, time lost due to alcohol-related illnesses by the 50 men in the sample was assessed from January 1967 to 31 December 1968 and was found to be a total of 2,758 days before and during counseling. By contrast, in the period after counseling from 1 January 1969 to 8 December 1970, only 250 days were lost by this group. The mean number of days lost was thus reduced to 5, compared with 55 before and during counseling. This latter figure includes the sick time incurred while each patient was hospitalized for detoxification and recovery at a halfway house. In addition, 42 men did not lose any time because of alcohol-related illnesses after counseling. Short-term sick leaves, reported by 15 men before and during treatment, were incurred by only 6 following treatment; long-term sick leaves (21 days or more) fell from 31 to 4 cases.

In order to determine the progress of these men four years after they had first been interviewed, in January 1973 we sent questionnaires to each member of the study group. Of the 50 men, 36 had remained on duty in the department, 30 on full and 6 on limited duty. All of these men responded and participated in the study. It was established that the remaining 14 men in the sample group had retired from active duty, and although questionnaires were sent to the addresses on their pension checks, none of them responded. Two had been dismissed and 12 had been retired for alcoholism-related physical disabilities.

From the 36-member group it was learned that 24 had maintained continuous sobriety, 11 had at least one "slip" (resumed drinking), and 1 had not stopped drinking. The abstinence of these 35 men had ranged from 2¼ to 4½ years. The "slips" averaged 3½ weeks, and those who slipped did so an average of two times. Continuous sobriety seemed to be correlated with attendance at AA meetings, for it was reported that 29 men continued to attend AA an average of twice a week; 18 men considered themselves active in AA, leading meetings, speaking frequently, and doing 12-step work assisting other alcoholics. There were 7 men hospitalized for alcoholism after being introduced to AA. Of the 36 men, 33 were married and living at home; 3 had been divorced because of drinking. The wives of 5 attended Alanon; none had children in Alateen.

Although the follow-up period was only four years after interview, the results should be meaningful to administrators of employee programs. The abstinent group, together with those who had early relapses but who are still working, comprise 70 percent of the entire group. This is a high recovery rate, but quite consistent with results reported by industrial programs.

A Summary of Statistics, 1966–74

Table 7.1 presents data on the experience of this program over a period of nine years, during which time 1,902 employees were interviewed as possible candidates for assistance with job-related problems. In more than one-fourth of these interviews the interviewer concluded that there was no problem, since the employee did not give evidence of having an immediate or serious problem with alcohol. These confrontations, however, did result in many referrals to marriage counselors, psychological services, AA meetings in the community, etc. Some of those interviewed were evidently not drinkers, but had been charged with intoxication by people arrested in the normal course of duty.

Also shown in the table are those who refused assistance when the counselor was convinced that a problem with alcohol really existed. The difficult judgment was made that such persons would be given more time to cooperate and referred to local AA meetings, and the commanding officer would be notified of their lack of cooperation. From the above two categories we had many subsequent returns for treatment, regretably in a more advanced stage of the illness, and some self-referrals seeking help in gaining greater insight into their alcohol problem.

These statistics seem cold and impersonal until one realizes that each person suffering from alcoholism touches the lives of 10 to 15 other people, including family, fellow workers, and the community in which he or she resides. While the figures do not show this, a large number of officers admitted to the program either had been of superior rank, or were promoted in rank and responsibility as a direct result of their recovery. An added benefit to the organization is the fact that recovered members frequently make referrals of their fellow employees in need of treatment. Table 7.1 does show, however, steady progress in reaching alcoholic employees within the New York City Police Department, with the majority of these employees returning to full duty with firearms.

With data compiled through 1974, we can compare the results of the service rendered in this program to those reported previously in the study of 50 men interviewed in 1967–68. In the first study, the men treated had an mean age of 37.4, with an average of 17 years of service and an alcohol problem of 9 years' duration before detection. Subsequent figures show a gradual lowering of the mean age at the time of admission to 34.9, and of the average years of service to 9.7. These figures suggest that the program is achieving earlier intervention into the problem-drinking cycle. Another hopeful indicator is an increase in voluntary

TABLE 7.1 STATISTICAL ANALYSIS OF NYCPD COUNSELING PROGRAM, 1966–1974

Year	*Initial Interview*	*No Problem*	*Refused Assistance*	*Returned to Full Duty*	*Therapy Carryover*	*Retired after 20 Years' Service*	*Surveyed* (Alcoholism)*	*Dismissed*	*Service Terminated*	*Died in Service*	*Resigned*
1966	165	41	14	25	69	6	7	2	0	0	1
1967	168	26	18	18	85	4	7	0	0	3	2
1968	133	20	6	50	33	7	7	1	2	2	4
1969	186	30	17	90	16	6	15	0	3	5	1
1970	307	101	27	114	31	5	9	2	2	3	13
1971	257	65	15	133	127	6	15	3	0	10	2
1972	220	100	12	86	74	10	5	0	0	12	3
1973	184	70	21	102	90	8	18	1	0	4	3
1974	282	142	29	111	90	5	8	9	0	4	1
Total	1,902	595	159	729	615	57	91	18	7	43	30

*Retired for disability.

admissions, with 28 men seeking help as self-referrals in 1974. The traditional cover-up and the stigma attached to a counseling operation may be finally yielding to a reputation in the Counseling Unit for credibility and effectiveness, with improved performance and personal well-being testifying to the success of the program.

Impact on Organizational Attitudes and Structure

Following the promulgation of the commissioner's policy, a gradual change of attitude toward the alcoholic employee resulted, primarily from supervisory training, orientation of police surgeons and the return of successful patients to the ranks.

Among the major changes are those governing disciplinary procedures for alcoholic officers. Before the inception of the formal Counseling Unit, men with medical problems were placed on a limited duty status and transferred from commands to clerical work in headquarters. In order to accommodate short-term illnesses such as alcoholism, temporary limited duty—wherein an officer is not transferred from his unit—has been established. Under this temporary limited duty, the commanding officer of the Medical Unit safeguards the patient's firearms, carries him on sick report while he is at the hospital and halfway house, and then removes him from the sick rolls and assigns him to headquarters for 90 days. At the end of 90 days, the chief surgeon then directs the man to return to his unit, leaving all administration to the Medical Unit and not to the Personnel Bureau.

On 7 January 1968 the *New York Times* (p. 72) published a report entitled "Twenty-nine Percent Fewer Policemen in City Suspended and Dismissed in 67." Part of the text reads as follows:

> 29% fewer policemen were suspended and dismissed from the New York Police Department in 1967 than in 1966. Statistics for the two years show that the number of policemen suspended had declined from 91 during 1966 to 64 during 1967.
>
> Acting Police Commissioner John Walsh said in an interview that he believes the decline in the number of suspensions and dismissals should be attributed to better trained and motivated men now serving in the department rather than to a slackening of enforcement efforts. . . . Commissioner Walsh said another explanation for the decline in formal disciplinary actions was that the department had been more successful in handling the problem of alcoholism.

We have also seen a steady reduction in fines in the trial room from 30 days' pay to 10 days' pay for intoxication. The supervision and cooperation of the sick employee has been assured by placing him on probation with the Counseling Unit for six months to one year. Here, disciplinary control aids the treatment plan with an added incentive for recovery—that of the threat of dismissal.

Another important improvement in attitude and organizational cooperation involves the recognition by administration of the disease of alcoholism. As the earlier study of 50 patients had shown, the department had attempted to handle alcoholism with discipline and not treatment. Suspensions were almost automatic in the cases of intoxication. Interim Order No. 32, dated 19 April 1974, which outlined causes for suspension, reflects the recent change in attitude on the part of the department. Section 3 of the order reads as follows: "A superior officer in charge of command *may* suspend a member of the department when the member is unfit for duty due to the effects of an intoxicant or drug aftereffects thereof."

Here is a great triumph for the behavioral aspect of administration, because in effect, when a member is willing to accept treatment at the Counseling Unit, he will not be suspended. He will not lose his job, medical coverage, or pension rights, and will remain on full pay while being treated. On the other hand, if a person is adamant and unwilling to accept any assistance, he might very well be suspended to force him to recognize what is a serious medical problem. Thus we find a specific change in the regulations which is entirely consonant with the police commissioner's policy as stated on page 7, paragraph 8: "Our primary purpose is to rehabilitate the alcoholic to a status of a sober, reliable, productive employee, thus retaining his skills, training, and experience."

CONCLUSION

Traditional personnel practices are now being shown to rest on concepts which no longer reflect the facts of organizational life. Bureaucratic theory, from which most of our traditional concepts of organizations have been derived, described organizations in mechanistic terms, viewing people primarily as a means for accomplishing work for organizational ends. These concepts were preoccupied with work assignments, division of labor, budgeting personnel, methods of analysis, and management technology for direction and control (Steggart 1971).

While all of us recognize the orderly, tight control of a bureaucratic organization as effective and efficient, especially in law enforcement agencies, still we are prodded by research in the behavioral sciences to believe that there are better ways to view superior-subordinate relationships that permit the exercise of managerial authority for the welfare of employees (Pfiffner and Presthus 1967, pp. 207–8). These behavioral concepts include concern for employee attitudes, expectations, value systems, and group tensions and conflicts, especially where they affect productivity and cohesion. The present tension and stress in police organizations is indicative of a breakdown of traditional theories' attempting to respond to modern aspects of employee stress. Police administrators should be more conscious of the dysfunctional consequences of traditional bureaucratic structure in a law enforcement agency. Argyris (1957, p. 233) maintains that often our traditional bureaucratic structures require behavior that tends to frustrate, cause conflict, and create failure for psychologically healthy individuals. Requiring men to work around the clock in tension-ladened areas of the city, relying solely on the ability of their brother officers to come to their aid in time of stress, often produces cynicism and defensive thinking on the part of police officers, forcing them at times even to break the law in order to defend what they consider justice. The remarkable factor here is not how many police officers become alcoholics, but rather why more police officers do not seek relief in alcohol in response to the tension and frustrations which they experience in their work.

We have presented this account of the Counseling Unit of the New York City Police Department as a modern approach to personnel practices—understanding the problem drinker as a sick person in need of help who can, with the proper treatment and supervision, become productive and properly adjusted within the work force. We feel that the employee has a right to care for medical problems, including alcoholism. The use of constructive coercion to motivate the alcoholic employee, however, does place a serious responsibility on agencies, first to provide the best medical care available when indicated and then to monitor the entire program of recovery: detoxification, medical care for other illnesses which may be present, halfway house, AA participation, and even psychological or psychiatric care for recidivists.

We hope that more and more administrators will become aware of and interested in helping the problem employee in order to assist and recover valuable, trained personnel. Many of us have heard AA members describe their efforts to stop drinking without any control or support from families or employers as "wasting 6 to 10 years before I saw the light." We feel that some coercion from the employer may well shorten this painful process. Police officers who defend our liberty, around the clock, in all our cities, should not be the last to receive treatment for alcoholism as a job-related illness: they should be among the first.

REFERENCES

American Medical Association. 1968. *Manual on Alcoholism.* Chicago: American Medical Association.

Argyris, C. 1957. *Personality and Organization.* New York: Harper.

Clinebell, H. J. 1968. *Understanding and Counseling the Alcoholic.* New York: Abingdon Press.

Dalton, M. 1959. *Men Who Manage,* New York: Wiley.

Dunne, J. A. 1973. "Counseling alcoholic employees in a municipal police department." *Quarterly Journal of Studies on Alcohol* 34:423–34.

Gerth, H. H., and C. W. Mills, eds. 1946. *From Max Weber: Essays in Sociology.* New York: Oxford University Press.

Hurwitz, J. I., and D. Lelos. 1968. "A multilevel interpersonal profile of employed alcoholics." *Quarterly Journal of Studies on Alcohol* 29:64–76.

Jellinek, E. M. 1946. "Phases in the drinking history of alcoholics: Analysis of a survey conducted by the official organ of Alcoholics Anonymous. *Quarterly Journal of Studies on Alcohol* 7:1–88.

Lippitt, G. L. 1969. *Organizational Renewal.* New York: Appleton-Century-Crofts.

Pfiffner, J. M., and R. Presthus. 1967. *Public Administration.* New York: The Ronald Press.

Steggart, F. X. 1971. "Organizational theory: Bureaucratic influences and the social welfare task." Address at Conference of Social Workers, New York.

Tiebout, H. M. 1965. "Crisis and surrender in treating alcoholism." *Quarterly Journal of Studies on Alcohol* 26:496–512.

Westley, W. A. 1951. "The police: A sociological study of law." Ph.D. dissertation, University of Chicago.

Wilcox, C. E. 1968. "The alcoholic in industry." *Ohio State Medical Journal* 64:78–82.

EIGHT / The Evaluation of Occupational Alcoholism Programs

RICHARD L. WILLIAMS and
JOSEPH TRAMONTANA

As is true of many other areas of applied research, it can be argued that the evaluation of occupational alcoholism or employee assistance programs[1] is still in its incipient stages. This statement is made for several reasons: there are insufficient empirical evaluations of current occupational alcoholism programs, making analytical comparisons difficult at best; the existing evaluations examine outcome within a narrow theoretical orientation rather than making a broad, empirical examination of impact; and the programs that have been evaluated have typically used different evaluative language and/or methodologies, resulting in incomparable findings (Williams and Temer 1975). Additionally, many of the attempts to investigate occupational programs have neglected the area of costs and benefits, with the result that few cost data are available, either to estimate the expenditures necessary to initiate or run a program or to serve as comparison experiences against which an existing program's cost effectiveness or efficiency could be evaluated.

Contributing to the underdevelopment of adequate program evaluation is the reluctance of many program directors to have their programs scrutinized. Williams and Temer (1975), on the basis of personal communications, have summarized some of the reasons stated by such directors. A few indicated that their program might be threatened by an objective evaluation; others claimed that evaluation might violate existing program confidentiality; and still others indicated that management had not requested this hard data.

Despite these limitations in current evaluation research in the field, it is apparent to us that evaluation of occupational alcoholism programs is essential to provide management the information necessary for intelligent program administration, decision-making, and direction. Accordingly, after a review of some of

1. The terms *occupational alcoholism program* and *employee assistance program* are used interchangeably in this chapter, although there are important differences between them (Wrich 1974).

the specific problems, we present a model that can serve as a useful framework for developing an empirical evaluation of an occupational alcoholism program. We have attempted to present rates, tables, and evaluation concepts that will be applicable to most programs, whether federal, state, local, or private, so that each may have a similar data base from which to operate.

FACTORS LIMITING THE ADEQUACY OF PROGRAM EVALUATIONS

In this section we review a number of biases and factors which, if not taken into account, may seriously limit the validity and comparability of research findings.

Sources of Bias in Alcoholism Treatment Research

Miller and associates (1970) have reviewed the research on alcoholism and have identified several sources of bias which frequently occur and which could invalidate conclusions of a study on an alcoholism program. Of the 34 outcome studies they reviewed, Miller et al. noted that less than one-half of them took these sources of bias into account when reporting their results. The authors concluded that those studies may represent a selected 5 percent of all alcoholics in the general population. Thus, principles emerging from studies of treatment which are thought to be generally applicable may in fact be relevant only to a very small segment of the population of interest. Because failure to report on sources of bias can have, and has had, very serious implications for the field of occupational alcoholism, the following discussion reviews the sources of bias identified by Miller et al. as they are often found in the literature on occupational alcoholism programs.

Different Definitions of Alcoholism. Differing definitions have historically prevented the direct comparison of alcoholism studies and continue to be a major problem for occupational alcoholism programs. The varied penetration and prevalence rates noted by different programs may be due solely to the different definitions of problem drinking and alcoholism. While it is unrealistic, given the nature of change in the field, to expect that common definitions will be arrived at quickly, each investigator should spell out the specific definition used in his program.

Biases in the Selection of the Treatment Population. The characteristics of a treatment population—such as occupational status, income level, and geographical area—may bear heavily upon the results of a program. Stanford Research Institute (SRI) issued a report (1975) on a follow-up study of clients at selected treatment centers (ATCs) funded by NIAAA and reported that "when client background is taken into account, ATCs have relatively uniform effects on outcome." It therefore appears advisable to equate client backgrounds and make group comparisons of these differences.

One source of bias in selection occurs when cases are drawn from special populations. The Comptroller General's estimate of a 1.5 percent prevalence of alcoholism in light industry compared with a 10 percent prevalence in heavy industry indicates the awareness of special populations (Comptroller General 1970). Clearly, if the treatment population is drawn exclusively from light industry, the results will apply only to similar populations.

Bias can also occur through selective referral. Occupational treatment programs often gain a reputation for servicing certain types of clients, with the result that only those types are referred. This means that the clients of a program are selected from and not necessarily representative of the total population. Those company programs which serve only blue-collar populations are examples of this type of selection. Similarly, if a program rejects a certain type of client, its results are applicable only to a portion of the problem-drinking population.

Sources of Bias in Reports of Program Success. Several sources of bias which may either overstate or understate success rates are often neglected in reports on program outcomes. One important example is refusal of referral. Aside from the fact that the characteristics and eventual outcomes of patients who refuse treatment have major implications for future programming, if a large number of referrals refuse treatment, the success of a program cannot be generalized to the total population for which it is intended.

Dropouts from treatment represent another source of potential bias. Dropouts include both those who are accepted for the program but drop out before treatment and those who drop out in the course of treatment. Again, these two groups may differ systematically from each other and from those who complete treatment. Often the droputs are ignored and the proportion not even reported. In presenting its results, SRI (1975) distinguished five categories of clients: contact only; pre-intakes; 30-day dropouts; 180-day dropouts; and stay-ins. Occupational programs could make the same kind of distinctions and add an additional category for those persons who are confronted by their supervisors but refuse treatment.

Clients in treatment are sometimes excluded from a study because of complicating factors, and this is not always reported. Current data on follow-up of the majority of clients in occupational programs is sketchy at best and indicates that many of the clients get "lost in the shuffle" from one treatment modality to another and are therefore excluded, at least for a period of time, from the proposed treatment. Additionally, some persons refuse to participate in follow-up, some change residences and cannot be located for follow-up, and clients who die before follow-up often cannot be rated in terms of improvement at the time of their discharge from the program. If these types of exclusions are not reported, the results could be erroneously assumed to apply to the total work force.

Problems in Relating Observed Outcomes to Program Intervention

In addition to the biases mentioned above which may invalidate industrial alcoholism research findings are a set of factors which, if not taken into account, may obscure the true impact of treatment on the observed outcome. While identified by Bergin (1971) as issues in adjudging the effectiveness of psychotherapy, these factors are equally applicable to industrial alcoholism treatment.

One such factor that must be addressed is the possibility of spontaneous recovery. Bergin's review of the psychotherapy literature on the number of persons who recover without formal treatment yielded estimates ranging from 0 to 52 percent, with an average of around 30 percent. Cahalan (1970) also reports on the recovery of problem drinkers without treatment intervention. Investigations into this phenomenon indicate that some of it may be self-generated and some of it may be due to informal treatment sources, either within the industrial setting or within the community, to which a person feels comfortable in turning for help in a time of stress and trouble. It should be remembered, therefore, that a certain proportion of those who improved during the course of a program would have gotten better anyway. The program cannot legitimately take credit for these individuals in computing its effectiveness. Until we are able to separate systematically spontaneous recoveries from the overall client population, cure or success rates should be evaluated and viewed as less than exact.

Related to the issue of spontaneous recovery is the problem of "regression effects." In many psychological and behavioral problem areas, a person does not seek help until he has reached a crisis. Within the supervisor confrontation situation, this may also be the case because the decision to confront an employee could be the result of the supervisor's having reached the last straw with that employee. A look at such an employee a week or two later might show him better regardless of treatment. The important point here is that any program dealing with desperate persons, or persons in an extreme state, will have its before-and-after estimates of effects of treatment contaminated by regression effects. Thus, absenteeism may decrease for a group placed in a treatment program, but it may also decrease for an identical group not getting treatment. To prove program effectiveness, improvement must be shown to result from treatment and not from such regression effects.

A final factor relating to the impact of treatment is the problem of "deterioration effects." This problem has been aptly stated by Edwards (1975): "If you have a treatment which is powerful enough to help some people, you will most likely be hurting a certain proportion of the persons who get the treatment. This is especially true in our present state of ignorance about the effects of different treatment on different types of people with different problems in different settings." Deterioration effects can so profoundly affect assessments of treatment effectiveness that many controlled outcome studies of psychotherapy show no significant mean differences between those who received treatment and those who did not (Bergin 1971).

Taking into account the effects of spontaneous recovery, regression, and deterioration, Bergin estimated the effectiveness of psychotherapy to be as follows: about 70 percent of patients get better, 20 percent show no change, and about 10 percent get worse. Since occupational alcoholism and employee assistance programs deal with similar behavioral disorders, we would expect to find similar phenomena, although the averages may be different and the rates may vary by type of industry, geographic location, guiding philosophy, or other factors.

Implications for Program Evaluators

Although unfortunate, it is often true that the more money a company expends on various troubled-employee programs, the more apt it will be to defend the success of that program (Williams and Moffat 1975). The directors of these employee assistance or occupational alcoholism programs have a much greater personal interest (their job) in the promotion of materials and evaluations that enhance the "successful" image of that program. Nevertheless, troubled-employee programs can better be justified on the basis of helping more people improve faster, or perhaps more easily, than by claiming miracles, dramatic personality changes, or sobriety. For example, if it were shown that an occupational alcoholism program helped 70 percent of those identified (Bergin 1971) get better a year sooner than they would have without the program, there would still be large savings to the company and to individuals and their families even though 20 percent of the patients stayed the same and 10 percent were worse off as a result of the intervention. Accordingly, the balance of this chapter is devoted to presenting a model for evaluating occupational programs that is aimed at yielding the most accurate and comparable estimates possible given the state of knowledge and techniques available to the field at present.

A MODEL FOR EVALUATING OCCUPATIONAL ALCOHOLISM PROGRAMS

The basic design for the model presented here was developed by a group of researchers at the University of Michigan School of Public Health (Deniston et al. 1968). Their model—which was developed to facilitate the planning, implementation, and evaluation of health programs—consists of a systematic and well-defined set of eight definitions of program attributes that can be readily adapted for use in evaluating occupational alcoholism programs (Edwards 1975).

Program Components

The first four terms in the model define a program, its goals, and the human and material resources available to it.

Program. The program is an organized response to reduce or eliminate one or more problems. This response includes (1) specification of one or more objectives, (2) selection and performance of one or more activities, and (3) acquisition and use of resources.

Objective. The objective is a situation or condition of people or of the environment which responsible personnel consider desirable to obtain. To permit subsequent evaluation, the statement of an objective must specify the nature of the situation or condition to be attained, the quantity or amount of the situation or condition to be attained, the particular group of people or portion of the environment in which attainment is desired, the geographic area of the program, and the time at or by which the desired situation or condition is intended to exist. Within this framework are three types of objectives. First, ultimate objectives are those which are desirable in and of themselves. Second, program objectives are those representing the outcome of implementing the program (e.g., identification and rehabilitation of 70 percent of the at-risk problem drinkers in a work force in a given year). And third, subobjectives are those objectives which must necessarily be achieved before the program objective(s) can be attained.

Activity. Activity is the work performed by program personnel and equipment in the service of an objective. *Activity,* as we use it, does not imply any fixed amount or scope of work; it may be applied with equal validity to such diverse efforts as writing a letter or providing comprehensive health care.

Resource. Resources are the personnel, funds, materials, and facilities available to support the performance of activity. Resources, like activities, may be described with varying levels of specificity.

Basic to the above formulation of a program is an emphasis on objectives. Many evaluation efforts are thwarted because the program's objectives have never been quantified. Historically, in the evaluation of occupational alcoholism programs, few people have asked, "Why does the program exist?" In talking to several of the program administrators of employee assistance or occupational alcoholism programs across the nation, Williams (1975) found that programs exist for many different reasons. Some directors state that their program is functioning because of its humanitarian value (e.g., it saves lives). Other, primarily community-oriented directors talk about the good public relations that the program affords the company with the community, as well as with the employees and their dependents. In contrast to the objectives of employers, unions often view a program as an alternative to dismissal. In other words, if the employee is referred to the program, the company should not fire him, at least, as long as the employee remains compliant within the expectations of the program. If, however, the employee is unable to complete the demands of the program successfully, then the usual grievance procedures may be filed. Although there is much talk throughout the literature about labor-management occupational alcoholism programs, it appears that often the program is either a *management* program or a *labor* program. Although several large companies have had sufficient cases before an arbitration board to develop standards of acceptance or rejection, it appears that the vast majority of programs have not reached this stage of development. Nevertheless, unions (particularly the UAW) are beginning to develop internal union programs and are cooperating with management in an effort to rehabilitate employees (Williams 1975).

Given the many different motivations that are possible among the parties involved in an occupational program, it may be necessary to work with program personnel to define the objectives in a measurable fashion. Although difficult, it is almost always possible to come up with some measurable indexes of program objectives, as does the model of Deniston, Rosenstock, and Getting. Moreover, some assessment must be made of resources and their utilization. Actual activity must be documented and subobjectives assessed. If this is done, weaknesses, trouble spots, and strengths in the program are readily apparent. In fully half of the evaluation efforts familiar to the authors, it has been discovered that activities have not actually been conducted as planned; and in most cases where this has occurred, the specified program objectives were not achieved.

Questions for Evaluation

The final four concepts in the model concern the types of questions that are necessary for program evaluation.

Appropriateness addresses the question, Is the program focused on important problems? Thus, appropriateness concerns the importance of the problem areas selected for programming and the relative emphasis or priority scheduled for their solution and/or eventual resolution. A variant of this question might be, Are our program objectives worthwhile and do they have a higher priority than other possible objectives of this or other programs?

Adequacy addresses the question, Is the program directed at all or only part of the problems? Objectives should be focused upon the resolution or alleviation of the situation(s) for which the program was developed. Several minor subobjectives, with quantifiable statements about how a problem might be reduced, may be more beneficial than a broad objective or "solution." The amount of the overall problem addressed by the objectives is a question of adequacy of program objectives. Detailed objectives for particular types of problems or persons experiencing these problems might prove more adequate in reaching specific target areas.

Effectiveness is defined as the number of objectives obtained because of the activities directed toward those objectives, and answers the question, How many of the predetermined objectives have been obtained?

Efficiency, defined as the total cost of obtaining the program objectives, asks, How much did it cost to get the degree of attainment observed?

Ideally, questions of appropriateness, adequacy, effectiveness, and efficiency should be asked prior to program implementation, so that data can be obtained for each conceptual area. However, the types of data and the issues involved are different for each of the four conceptual areas, and it is of primary importance, therefore, that the distinction between them and their related evaluative questions be kept separate.

Because obtaining answers to the question of program effectiveness is often the most complex area of evaluation, the following two sections explore in detail the considerations involved in designing studies and in developing frequency rates for assessing effectiveness. Then, using the model outlined in this section, an employee assistance program for problem drinkers is evaluated in terms of appropriateness, adequacy, effectiveness, and efficiency.

DESIGNS FOR EVALUATING THE EFFECTIVENESS OF OCCUPATIONAL ALCOHOLISM PROGRAMS

In industrial alcoholism programs the primary objective is most often to effect a change in the job performance of problem-drinking employees. Consequently, as with applied psychological research in general, evaluating program effectiveness involves the measurement of behavior change. The basic designs for evaluating the effectiveness of industrial alcoholism programs are outlined in Table 8.1. As will be discussed below, the levels indicated in the table represent ascending complexities of design. Unfortunately, many applied evaluation efforts have not been attempted because of the view that a study without rigorous controls (levels 5 and 6) is worthless. It is not always possible, however, to start evaluation at highly complex levels, and "good applied research has to evolve over time" (Edwards 1975). Moreover, certain checks and precautions can be taken to offset some of the limitations inherent in the less sophisticated forms of design, and these will be indicated.[2]

What Happened? (Or, What Is Happening?)

The primary question of "What happened?" is typically answered in one of two ways. The first is to examine individual cases, either for a testimonial or "expert" assertion to determine the effect of an occurrence, or through a more detailed case investigation. Although the testimonial method often yields insightful information, it is a subjective approach; and replication or further examination of the data is limited. Consequently, case studies, in which a wealth of information is presented on the progression of the drinking problem and the resolution which is or is not achieved, are frequently used as a clinical method for describing what happened in individual cases. Both the testimonial and case approaches are usually used at level 1 or level 2 designs (Table 8.1). Level 1 (0)

2. The section which follows is extracted from Edwards' earlier model on evaluation (1975). Additional comments reflected in recent research have been inserted by the present authors where relevant and may completely change the scope or intent presented by the original author.

TABLE 8.1 DESIGNS USED FOR EVALUATION

Question	*Level*	*Design**
What happened?	1.	0
	2.	$X \rightarrow 0$
How much happened?	3.	$0 \rightarrow X \rightarrow 0$
	4.	$000 \rightarrow X \rightarrow 000$
How much happened compared with doing something else?	5.	$0 \rightarrow X_1 \rightarrow 0$ (The treatment group)
		$0 \rightarrow X_2 \rightarrow 0$ (The different treatment group)
How much happened compared with doing nothing?	6.	$0 \rightarrow X \rightarrow 0$ (The treatment group)
		0 (The no-treatment group)

*0 = evaluation of subject; X = some form of treatment.

would involve descriptions of individuals and a detailed write-up of what happened from the examiner's view. At level 2 ($X \rightarrow 0$), some treatment (X) is administered, and for each case a writeup is made describing what happened.

Because of the focus on individual cases and because of the quantity of information—some relevant and some irrelevant—that is presented, the testimonial and case study methods cannot yield a good, overall picture of program effectiveness. An additional problem involved in the study of individual cases—observer bias—can be offset by the use of multiple observers and of reliability and validity checks expanded on by Herman and Tramontana (1971). These checks, which are basic to any single-subject or same-subject designs in which individuals are being compared with themselves, are as follows:

Interrater agreement. Two observers evaluate or rate the same subjects simultaneously but independently. The reliability check involves computing the percentage of agreements per subject per rating period as compared with the total number of observations.

Naïve rater. Since raters who are aware of the experimental goals may reach a high level of agreement and be biased in their ratings, utilization of a naïve and independent rater who knows nothing about the experimental goals or about which subjects belong in each comparison group decreases the possibility of such experimental bias.

Time-sampling validity check. If time samples of behavior are used as dependent variables, there is the need to check the validity of the assumption that the behavior observed at fixed spacings in time adequately represents the behavior occurring during the entire experimental session. To accomplish this, randomly chosen subjects can be observed on a continuous basis by one experimenter while the other is engaged in the regular time-sampling procedure. A correlation coefficient can then be computed between the time sample and continuous sample to give the experimenters an estimate of the validity of their time-sampling technique.

A second way of answering the question of what happened is to examine a population of alcoholic or problem-drinking employees. Here too, level 1 or level 2 designs may be used. At level 1—observation only (0)—one might look at the population of a plant during a specified period and determine the number of problem drinkers and the percentage of them who kept or lost their jobs. In the early literature on the extent of the problem of alcoholism in industry, most studies were of this variety. With the growth of industrial alcoholism programs, however, designs at level 2 have become common, whereby an evaluation of the population of problem drinkers following treatment ($X \rightarrow 0$) is made to determine the percentage who improved as a result of the program. The deficiency in level 1 and level 2 designs is that there is no comparison group to control for passage of time, extraneous variables, etc.

How Much Happened?

This question asks not only "What happened?" but also tries to quantify or measure the degree of accomplishment or change. The designs at levels 3 and 4 of Table 8.1 are most commonly used to evaluate this question. In these designs, evaluations or observations are made both before and after the treatment. The level 4 design is called the extended time series design and employs multiple observations to show the stability or the trends in the behavior both before and after treatment.

An example of this type of pre-post design was obtained from the evaluation of the East Carolina University's National Occupational Alcoholism Training Institute. At the beginning and end of the three-week training program, the trainees were asked to indicate how much they felt they knew about the various roles of industry in generating solutions for problem drinking. On a five-point rating scale, the mean score for the 101 trainees that answered was 2.8 at the beginning, and 3.3 at the end of training, a difference that was statistically significant. Additionally, on the pre-test, 35 percent of the respondents said they had "none" or "very little" knowledge, while on the post-test, only 12 percent fell into the two bottom categories of the five-point scale. Thus, using this pre- and post-test design, it was possible to show not only a nonchance change in perceived knowledge (what happened), but also the amount of the change (how much happened) as a result of training. However, it may be argued that the trainees, because of biases and expectancies, would rate their knowledge higher in post-testing, regardless of the content or value of the training session. For this reason, the designs at levels 5 and 6 provide more meaningful evaluation data.

How Much Was Accomplished Compared with Doing Something Else (or Nothing)?

The designs at levels 5 and 6 add the new element of a group that receives a different treatment (level 5) or a group that receives no treatment (level 6). An example of a level 5 design would be a comparison of the scores of employees treated in a company's in-house alcoholism program (treatment group) with those of employees treated in a community-based program. A level 5 design answers the question, "How much was accomplished compared with doing something else?" A level 6 design answers the question, "How much was accomplished compared with doing nothing?" Level 5 and 6 designs may be of two types: the pre-test–post-test comparison group design or the pre-test–post-test control group design. In the first instance, there is no way to determine whether the two groups (i.e., treatment and other or no-treatment) are similar, whereas in the control group design, the groups are matched so that they will be as similar as possible. The comparison group design is not as strong as the control group design, since measured differences may reflect differences between the two groups (e.g., age, occupation) beyond the impact of treatment.

The ideal design for evaluating program effectiveness would be a pre-test–post-test, no-treatment control group design. Such a design is the epitome of empirical research and a basic design for experimental studies. It allows the evaluator to answer not only the questions of "What happened?" and "How much happened?" but also the question of "How much happened compared to doing nothing?" This is extremely important because, as the results of Cahalan's (1970) work indicate, most problem drinkers change their drinking patterns within three years without benefit of treatment. What then must be investigated is not whether a person is helped by the program, but how much and how soon he is helped compared with predicted change without intervention. A pre-test–post-test control group design would allow the researcher to say whether or not any change observed was greater than what would have occured without treatment, in addition to whether or not the change was large enough to be a non–chance finding. Unfortunately, the control group design is seldom found in applied research. Indeed, the authors were unable to find a single study of an occupational alcoholism program that used a matched control group.

More common in the literature is the comparison group design, used either with a group which is exposed to different treatment or one which receives no treatment. An example of the comparison group design was also presented by the National Occupational Alcoholism Training Institute, although it is not a pre-test–post-test design. Five months after the three-week initial training program, a follow-up workshop was held. Ninety-one of the original participants attended, along with 19 new persons who had not attended the training program. At the beginning of the workshop, participants were again asked how much they felt they knew about the various roles of industry in developing solutions to problem drinking. The mean scores of the trainees and of the comparison group were significantly different. If it could be assumed that the two groups were basically similar, one could conclude that the training experience led to a significantly greater perceived knowledge than did no training experience. However, uncontrolled factors could also be responsible for the observed difference, and so the evidence only suggests that the training program produced the difference. Had a control group been used and the same difference been observed, then a stronger conclusion could be possible.

While the above discussion points to the pre-test–post-test no-treatment control group design as the most desirable for measuring behavior change, and thus for evaluating program effectiveness, "no systematic effort to randomly assign alcoholic employees to occupational programs, on the one hand, and to leave them alone group on the other, has been attempted" (Roman and Trice 1976). Although typical psychological experiments use, as a measure of change, the difference in performance between a group that has been exposed to the experimental variable and a control group that has not been exposed, applied research often precludes such experimental manipulation (Tramontana 1970). For example, it may be difficult and/or questionable to offer counseling to one group of employees and withhold it to another (control) group. There is also a problem of using nonvolunteers as a control group, since nonvolunteers are frequently different in many ways from volunteers.

Therefore, a frequently used experimental procedure is a single-subject (or same-subject) design referred to by Sidman (1960) as "stable state research."

One immediate virtue of the stable state as a substitute for the control group is a reduction in the statistical effects of intersubject variability. The stable state procedure increases enormously the sensitivity of the behavioral measurements. Variables that might be dismissed as having little or no effect when group comparisons are made may prove to be extremely significant when evaluated against an individual's own stable baseline.

One of the most frequently employed designs in stable state research involves the so-called ABAB design: (A) baseline, (B) treatment, (A2) return to baseline or reversal of contingencies, and (B2) reinstatement of treatment conditions. While the ABAB design is the more scientifically sound, some applied (nonexperimental) situations make reversal of contingencies undesirable, and thus ABA designs (corresponding to level 3 in Table 8.1) are utilized. Whatever the stable state design used, the individual is compared with his own stable baseline (which may be stably unstable—i.e., with regular "peaks and valleys"). The utility of data in this type of research depends not so much on ultimate stability as on the reliability and validity of the criterion. That is, if the experimental manipulation of steady states, as defined by the criterion measures, yields data that are orderly and that represent functional relations which are replicable, the experimental design adequately tests the hypotheses it purports to test—in this case, that occupational programs improve an individual's drinking habits and decrease his job deficiencies related to those habits. The problem of developing consistent, valid, and measurable criteria of behavior change is considered in the following section.

FREQUENCY RATES FOR EVALUATING PROGRAM EFFECTIVENESS

One of the earliest sets of rates for measuring effectiveness of occupational programs included measures of impaired productivity, interpersonal friction, absenteeism, and costs of health and accident problems (Winslow et al. 1966). These rates have been extended and clarified by several researchers (Williams 1975; Schlenger and Hayward 1975; Roman and Trice 1976), and in addition to the above criteria of behavior change, measures of program effectiveness have come to include the extent to which the program is reaching a specified target population. While the use of such rates is gaining a wide acceptance among program personnel, they have been applied and interpreted inconsistently, and often with a lack of specificity. For example, when an administrator talks about absenteeism, he usually does not specify whether it is on the job, off the job, or even job-related. Many programs refer to health costs and insurance costs as though they were closely related, although this has yet to be actuarially demonstrated (Williams and Temer 1975).

In this section the literature on the use of rates for evaluating program effectiveness is reviewed, and some modifications to resolve earlier discrepancies are suggested. Should people begin to use the same rates, it will become easier to evaluate programs and share meaningful experiences, methodology, and data. We assume that geographical, cultural, social, and industrial differences exist, and that by using the rates developed below, we may be able to generate data to document such differences. As discussed in the preceding section, it is of particular importance from an evaluation perspective that each of the above rates be compared with those applying to a control group of similar persons within the same organization who are not involved in the program. If for some reason it is not possible to match control groups, the population norm(s) of the organization should be used. If organizational population norms are used, they should be clearly stated and the methods for determining them should be specified (Williams and Temer 1975).

Sickness

The sickness frequency rate is computed by taking the total number of sick days and dividing it by the total number of persons in an organization. We define sick days as those days on which a person reports in sick or on which medical services are necessary (Williams and Temer 1975). Several companies have reported experiences with sickness frequency rates. Illinois Bell reports a significant reduction in the number of sickness disability cases within their program: "Five years before the program began, the number of sickness disability cases (more than seven days of reported illness) for the persons in the program was 662. Five years after program intervention, this total number of cases had dropped to 356 for those persons participating in the program" (Asma 1975). The Boston Edison Company reports that among 196 employees referred to a program, there had been approximately 116 hospitalizations for both the employees themselves and/or members of their families because of alcoholism. In the five-year period following their admission to the program, however, hospitalizations averaged 24 per year, with the average period of hospitalization being 15 days (Ravin 1975). The occupational alcoholism program within the New York City Police Department reports that the average number of sick days used before counseling was 35, but dropped to 16.8 days in the year following return to work. The New York City Police Department further reports that a total of 250 days were lost by the group after counseling in comparison to 2,758 days before and during counseling. Short-term sick leaves were reduced from 15 men before and during treatment to 6 men following treatment (Dunne 1975).

One of the primary things we noticed in reviewing the literature is that the basis for determining the sickness frequency rate varies from program to program. *Every* sick day should be counted and not just those that exceed a given limit (i.e., five days, seven days, etc.). Until a program has reached the stage of development wherein *all* absenteeism due to sickness is reported as it occurs, it will be difficult to determine whether a sickness frequency rate for those persons with drinking problems is different from those without drinking problems (Williams 1975).

Absenteeism

The absenteeism frequency rate is the rate most often used and probably the most misunderstood of all rates employed today by occupational alcoholism or employee assistance programs. The absenteeism frequency rate should be determined by dividing the number of days absent by the total number of persons within an employed population. This particular rate measures only *off*-the-job absenteeism. The only semiempirical study of an on-the-job absenteeism rate that we reviewed was developed by Williams and Lindley (1975), wherein a mean is determined between the clients' and supervisors' rating of on-the-job performance impairment by a neutral third party. The absenteeism frequency rate should address itself to both on-the-job and off-the-job absenteeism patterns (Trice and Roman 1972).

The absenteeism rate is extremely difficult to relate to occupational alcoholism programs because of many confounding variables. People will be absent for the oddest reasons, and in fact, some feel that they have not received all their benefits unless they have used every available sick day allowed them by the company. Indeed, some companies and state offices allow absenteeism until it has reached the limit, or norm, for that employed group. "However, gross group differences appear to exist between the employed population at large and those persons with drinking problems" (Trice and Roman 1972). Consequently, occupational alcoholism programs do offer the potential for developing data on problems secondary to problem drinking (e.g., marital, legal, financial) that may have a direct effect on absenteeism. It is important that such data be corrected for alcohol relatedness to demonstrate the alcohol-related absenteeism rate as well as for purposes of secondary prevention and early case finding in problem drinking and alcoholism (Williams and Temer 1975).

Turnover

The turnover frequency rate (usually calculated yearly) may be one of the most interesting factors in occupational programming because of the relationship of alcoholism to termination, disabling accidents, voluntary and forced resignations, and death. The turnover frequency rate is computed by dividing the total number of persons who have left the company (resigned, quit, fired, etc.) by the total number of persons within the organization (Williams and Temer 1975). There appear to be conflicting data relative to turnover rates associated with problem drinking (Cahalan 1970). Roman and Trice (1976) report that problem-drinking employees are not characterized by high rates of turnover. We recognize that there are many factors associated with turnover. However, while it is rarely reported in the literature, because of its importance to the field it should be measured. It may be constructive to continue computation of such base data until sufficient information is gathered to assess the total impact of problem drinking upon turnover.

Accidents

The accident disability rate is self-explanatory and has been well documented in programs such as those described above, notably Illinois Bell and the INSIGHT Program at Kennecott Copper (Asma 1975; Jones 1975). The accident disability rate is computed by dividing the days of disability by the total number of persons within an organization (Williams and Temer 1975). This rate has also produced conflicting data. Trice and Roman (1972) reported that problem-drinking employees do not show an exceptional number of on-the-job accidents. Another investigator (Brenner 1967), however, found that problem drinkers do show high rates of off-the-job accidents.

Referrals

The referral rate is the rate by which people are referred to an occupational alcoholism or employee assistance program. It is important to distinguish three basic types of referral rates: the overall referral rate, the self-referral rate, and the coerced referral rate. The total referral rate is defined as the total number of referrals divided by the total number of persons within the organization (Williams and Temer 1975). The self-referral rate is the number of self-referrals divided by the total number of persons within an organization. The coerced referral rate is the number of involuntary referrals (supervisor-coerced) divided by the total number of persons within an organization.

The self-referral and coerced referral rates are expected to give an indication of how well a program is being accepted by those for whom it is intended: the better the program is functioning, the higher the self-referral rate will be. Several programs receive a high percentage of self-referrals and indicate that this is due in part to the educational, training, and promotional efforts of the individuals in charge of the program (Williams and Temer 1975).

Although the literature indicates that absenteeism and referrals in program development are inversely related, this does not always appear to be true. There are programs that we have reviewed that have had an ever-increasing absenteeism rate despite an increase in number of referrals to the company employee assistance program. Therefore, number of referrals cannot stand alone as a measure of success without corroborative success indices.

Health Costs

Health, medical, and surgical rates have been documented in programs such as INSIGHT at Kennecott Copper and those of several other large organizations. The INSIGHT program reports a 55.35 percent decrease in health, medical, and surgical costs after individual participation in the company program (Jones 1975). We define the health rate as the total amount of money expended by the company/state on its employees within one calendar year for health costs as provided for in the insurance policy of that company or state. We are well aware that many individuals will spend money outside the insurance system for health care and that these costs may not be accounted for.

People Problems

The people problem rate is the frequency of particular types of problems as reported to the employee assistance program. It is defined as the number of people having a given type of problem (familial, alcohol, marital, psychological, legal, etc.) divided by the total number of persons within the organization. This entire area has yet to be evaluated systematically. Once the frequency and types of people problems have been determined for a program, they may then be compared individually for the above rates. We feel that there will be differences in each of the types of people problems reported and that these differences should be taken into account for planning purposes.

Penetration

The penetration rate for alcohol-related problems is defined as the total number of alcohol and alcohol-related referrals divided by the at-risk population. The definition of the at-risk population is that determined by Cahalan (1970) as modified by Marden (1975). This penetration rate differs from that typically presented in the literature because it includes only individuals referred for alcoholism or alcohol-related problems, as opposed to the number of persons within a program divided by a percentage of persons within the organization. Although this latter total penetration rate might be useful in determining the percentage of persons referred to a program, it may have little or nothing to do with problem drinking or alcoholism (Williams 1975).

Schlenger and Hayward (1975) have refined the penetration-rate computation process in an empirical manner as follows:

$$\text{Penetration Rate} = \frac{PD_I}{PD_W},$$

where PD_I = number of problem drinkers identified and referred to treatment by the program during a given time period

PD_W = number of problem drinkers in the organization's work force during a given time period.

The numerator of the penetration rate is relatively straightforward; however, the denominator is not so easily determined. Since the actual number of problem drinkers in the work force is never known with certainty, penetration rates are usually computed using an estimate of prevalence as the denominator:

$$PD_W = AE,$$

where A = estimated proportion of problem drinkers in the work force

E = number of employees.

The difficulty with such an approach is that prevalence estimates vary widely. Additionally, ascertaining the number of employees is not so simple as it might at first seem. Since the penetration rate is computed for a specified period of time, the number of employees should be the total number of persons employed during that time period. In other words, it should be the number of persons employed at the beginning of the period plus those hired during the period. This provides an accurate reflection of the *total* working population from which program clients could have been identified. Thus, for the first year of operation, the accurate formula for estimating program penetration may be expressed as

$$\text{Penetration Rate} = \frac{PD_I}{A(E+H)},$$

where PD_I = number of problem drinkers identified and referred to treatment during the time period
A = the estimated proportion of problem drinkers in the work force
E = number of employees at the beginning of the time period
H = number of employees hired during the time period

An additional problem arises, however, in computing the penetration rate for subsequent time periods. This problem stems from the fact that the estimate of the number of problem drinkers in the work force must be adjusted because some of the company's problem drinkers have already been identified and referred to treatment—that is, the estimated 6 to 10 percent who are problem drinkers (among employed persons) in populations without a program. As the program identifies and helps problem drinkers, some adjustments must be made in the prevalence estimate to take this into account. Thus, as years go by and persons pass through and are helped by the program, the estimated prevalence of problem drinking should be reduced. Stated simply, as one makes progress toward solving a problem, the size of the problem is reduced. Thus, in the second and subsequent years, the penetration rate formula should be adjusted as follows:

$$\text{Penetration Rate} = \frac{PD_I}{A(E+H) - C},$$

where C = the number of persons who are successfully treated and retain their jobs (Schlenger and Hayward 1975).

APPLICATION OF THE EVALUATION MODEL

This section presents an evaluation of Occupational Health Services (OHS), a private corporation in Alameda County, California, which provides occupational health services to the county in the form of an employee assistance program for problem drinkers and their dependents. OHS is an interdisciplinary group of medical, behavioral, engineering, and administrative personnel dedicated to the promotion and maintenance of a positive state of organizational and individual health and well-being. The corporation is contracted with the Alameda County Health Care Services Agency to assist organizations in determining the value and format of an employee assistance program based upon their particular needs; assist in the development of a policy statement regarding the program; provide training for management, supervisors, and stewards; assist in the education of employees regarding the program; provide initial counseling, problem identification, and goal setting for troubled employees; provide professional and preprofessional referral and treatment guidelines; provide follow-up and direct consultation with employees and management; and assist in the analysis of benefits available from insurance coverage.

In June 1975, the senior author reached an agreement with the president of OHS, Mr. Robert Temer, to evaluate the program using the model discussed within this chapter. The program had been functioning as a demonstration to determine effectiveness, efficiency, and costs for a period of six months; and the figures and percentages derived are for that period of time only. Although much of the base-rate data were not available at that time, sufficient information was provided by OHS and Alameda County personnel to use the basic evaluation model and provide a tentative assessment of services to date.

Appropriateness

The occupational alcoholism program is the priority program within OHS, taking precedence over the other services OHS provides to the employed population of Alameda County. The five persons constituting the full-time staff devote approximately 95 percent of their time to the occupational alcoholism program. One full-time staff member is assigned to administration, one to secretarial duties, one to employee counseling, and two to programs development, although there is occasional overlap of function and responsibility. In addition, a supplemental staff of 20 consultants provides expertise as needed in such areas as developing alcoholism awareness, supervisory training, medical and psychological counseling services, systems analysis, and value clarification.

The prevalence of problem drinking by the employed population of Alameda County was determined to be 8 percent, using NIAAA's estimated average (Marden 1975). The civilian employed population in Alameda County was 454,500 as of July 1972. Median family income (Bureau of the Census 1970) was reported to be $11,600. Total gross income from employment in Alameda County was $3,830,980,500. Estimated economic loss attributable to reduced job performance by troubled employees was estimated to be $76.5 million annually (Comptroller General 1970). Direct contract cost for the initiation of an occupational alcoholism program was $80,000 annually. Penetration of the population at risk was targeted for maximum effect at 5 percent (considered the optimal penetration goal), and a savings of $4,640,000 annually was estimated at this penetration level.

Adequacy

Based upon scheduled staff counseling time and anticipated referrals at the .02 and .05 level, the estimated capacity of the occupational alcoholism program was stated in the OHS contract with Alameda County to be an employed population of approximately 10,000 persons annually. The size of the problem using an 8 percent at-risk figure for an employed group of 454,500 is 36,360 employees. The counseling capacity of the program makes services available for an employed population of 25,700 persons. This figure exceeds the projected program capacity by 250 percent.

Effectiveness

The effectiveness of the OHS program during the period of evaluation is determined, according to the model, by measuring the proportion of objectives achieved.

Objective 1 was to develop awareness of the cost and extent of alcohol abuse among a select group of 17,000 employees (of employers expressing interest) in Alameda County. In order to develop awareness, OHS conducted a campaign of direct mail, newspaper, and radio advertising. Approximately 29 companies are in some developmental stage of occupational programming. Ten companies, with an employed population of 16,500 persons, and the County of Alameda, with 9,200 employees, have developed functional occupational alcoholism programs as a direct result of OHS program consultations. The employed population that now has occupational programs available is 25,700. Each of these employees directly affects an estimated three other persons, for a total penetration of the population of Alameda County of 102,800 persons.

Objective 2 was to encouarge acceptance and encourage the development of an occupational alcoholism program by 1,400 large employers in Alameda County. Each of the 1,400 industries/companies within Alameda County with 25 or more employees was informed of the services provided by OHS by mail or personal contact. Included with the letter was an attitude questionnaire for the companies to fill out and return. OHS received a 3.7 percent return rate on the questionnaire. Also included was an invitation to a seminar entitled ''Problem Drinking/

Alcoholism: A Legitimate Labor-Management Affair." Of the initial 1,400 invited, 60 persons attended the seminar.

Objective 3 was to provide direct occupational alcoholism services to a select portion of the 15,600 small businesses in Alameda County. The provision of occupational alcoholism programs for small businesses (fewer than 25 employees) has characteristically proven difficult nationally as well as in California. The above-mentioned seminar was prominently advertised in the two principal newspapers of Alameda County. Additionally, two radio stations were utilized for a period of two days to advertise the seminar and the occupational alcoholism programs to all citizens in the county. As a result of the advertising, five inquiries were received from employers with 100 or fewer employees. One of the persons inquiring employed fewer than 25 persons and was not interested in establishing a program.

Objective 4 was to develop an occupational alcoholism program for Alameda County's employees and their families. At the time of evaluation, the program was approximately 80 percent completed. A policy statement had been developed, employee awareness had been fostered via direct mail to the employees, one person within the county had been designated as coordinator of the program, and referrals (the majority are self-referrals) were using the pretreatment counseling services of OHS. The county program, though functioning, should begin an internal evaluation process that can only be instituted within the program at a county personnel level. Although the supervisory training process has begun and has reached approximately 100 supervisors, the training process should be accelerated for maximum impact and increased effectiveness with the remaining 800 supervisors.

Objective 5 was to provide assistance to attempt to reach 5 percent of the at-risk employed population of Alameda County and/or their dependents suffering from personal problems (alcoholism) that may affect job performance. OHS has seen or been contacted by 191 persons within the last six months. This represents a penetration rate of 13 percent of the 1,374 at-risk troubled employees within Alameda County for whom OHS has developed occupational alcoholism programs. Since OHS, in its role as programmer and pretreatment counselor, does not have access to personnel records that would enable it to determine the effect of treatment once a referral has been made, these measures need to be developed by the responsible county or company representative utilizing the occupational program.

Objective 6 was to attempt to demonstrate and achieve a cost savings for Alameda County. As stated above, OHS has been contacted by 191 employed persons or their families. Assuming that 70 percent of these individuals have been helped (Bergin 1971), the net savings to Alameda County would be \$388,600. These figures are determined by using a 70 percent improvement rate × 25 percent improvement in impairment × \$11,600 yearly median family income (Comptroller General 1970). This represents a return of \$5.65 for each dollar spent by Alameda County for the employee assistance program.

Efficiency

The cost in resources to obtain the stated objectives can be summarized as follows:

Resources: \$80,000 per contract with Alameda County
Percentage of resources available: 100 percent
Percentage of stated goals attained:

1. Developing awareness: 20 percent of county employed population
2. Developing programs: 5.6 percent of total employed population
3. Contacting 1,400 industries: 100 percent complete
4. Developing programs in small companies: 100 percent contacted, but none currently interested
5. Occupational alcoholism program for Alameda County: 80 percent completed
6. Penetration of at-risk population: 13 percent

Cost savings to Alameda County: \$388,600.

The distribution of the \$80,000 of the original contract with Alameda County among the above-stated goals was \$8,000 each for objectives 1 and 2, and \$16,000 for objectives 3 through 6. The relative cost per attainment of the six goals is outlined below.

1. Developing awareness by 102,000 employees and dependents of occupational alcoholism programs: \$0.07 per person
2. Developing 10 programs for 16,500 employees: \$0.48 per employee
3. Contacting 1,400 large industries with an employee population of 302,873 to develop programs: \$0.05 per employee
4. Contacting and promoting occupational alcoholism programs for 15,600 small companies (151,637 employees): \$0.10 per employee
5. Developing occupational alcoholism programs for 9,200 county employees and dependents (27,600 persons): \$0.58 per person

6. Reaching and providing pretreatment counseling of troubled employees (191 persons): $83.77 per employee

Recommendations

On the basis of the evaluation of the OHS occupational alcoholism program, several recommendations were made:

—Review and initiate tasks not yet completed by the county/companies, including an information system for program evaluations; procedures for the routine and periodic collection of client and staff ratings of status for each client; follow-up procedures; and procedures for the collection of absenteeism, accident, health, and grievance costs.
—Increase budget and programming staff. Target population of 10,000 employees has been exceeded by 250 percent.
—Increase counseling pretreatment staff to handle growing client-coerced and self-referrals.
—Continue development of programs with employers of 25 or more persons only. This development will necessitate completing the second and third points above.
—Continue training of county supervisors. A single mass training effort is recommended for maximum effectiveness and efficiency.
—Continue special seminars for the "gatekeepers" (judges, clergy, police, etc.) on special-funds basis.

REFERENCES

Asma, F. E. 1975. "Long-term experience with rehabilitation of alcoholic employees." In R. Williams and G. Moffat, eds., *Occupational Alcoholism Programs*. Springfield, Ill.: Charles C Thomas.

Bergin, A. E. 1971. "The evaluation of therapeutic outcomes." In A. L. Bergin and S. L. Garfield, eds., *Handbook of Psychotherapy in Behavior Change: An Empirical Change*. New York: Wiley.

Brenner, B. 1967. "Alcoholism and fatal accidents." *Quarterly Journal of Studies on Alcohol* 28:517–27.

Cahalan, D. 1970. *Problem Drinkers: A National Survey*. San Francisco: Jossey-Bass.

Comptroller General of the United States. 1970. *Substantial Cost Savings from Establishment of Alcoholism Programs for Federal Civilian Employees*. Report to the Special Subcommittee on Alcoholism and Narcotics of the Committee on Labor and Public Welfare, U.S. Senate. Washington, D.C.: U.S. Government Printing Office.

Deniston, O. L., I. N. Rosenstock, and V. A. Getting. 1968. "Evaluation of program effectiveness." *Public Health Reporter* 83:323–35.

Dunne, J. A. 1975. "Counseling the alcoholic employee in a municipal department." In R. L. Williams and G. H. Moffat, eds., *Occupational Alcoholism Programs*. Springfield, Ill.: Charles C Thomas.

Edwards, D. W. 1975. "The evaluation of troubled-employee and occupational alcoholism programs." In R. L. Williams and G. H. Moffat, ed., *Occupational Alcoholism Programs*. Springfield, Ill.: Charles C Thomas.

Herman, S. H., and J. Tramontana. 1971. "Instructions and group versus individual reinforcement in modifying disruptive group behavior." *Journal of Applied Behavior Analysis* 4:113–19.

Jones, O. 1975. "Insight: A program for troubled people." In R. L. Williams and G. H. Moffat, eds., *Occupational Alcoholism Programs*. Springfield, Ill.: Charles C Thomas.

Marden, P. G. 1975. *A Procedure for Estimating the Potential Clientele of Alcoholism Service Programs*. Prepared for the Division of Special Treatment and Rehabilitation Programs, NIAAA.

Miller, B. A., A. D. Porkney, J. Valles, and S. E. Cleveland. 1970. "Bias sampling in alcoholism treatment research." *Quarterly Journal of Studies on Alcohol* 31:97–107.

Ravin, I. S. 1975. "Formulation of an alcoholism rehabilitation program at Boston Edison Company." In R. L. Williams and G. H. Moffat, eds., *Occupational Alcoholism Programs*. Springfield, Ill.: Charles C Thomas.

Roman, P. M., and H. M. Trice. 1976. "Alcohol abuse and work organizations." In B. Kissen and H. Begleiter, eds., *The Biology of Alcoholism,* vol. 4, pp. 445–517. New York: Plenum Press.

Schlenger, W. E., and B. J. Hayward. 1975. "Occupational programming: Problems in research and evaluation." Paper presented at the International Meeting of the Alcohol and Drug Association of North America, Chicago.

Sidman, M. 1960. *Tactics of Scientific Research: Evaluating Experimental Data in Psychology*. New York: Basic Books.

Stanford Research Institute. 1975. *Summary, Conclusions, and Recommendations, Excerpted from Final Report: A Follow-Up Study of Clients at Selected Alcoholism Treatment Centers Funded by NIAAA*. Menlo Park, Calif.

Tramontana, J. 1971. "A review of research on behavior modification in the home and school." *Educational Technology* 11:61–64.

Trice, H. M., and P. M. Roman. 1972. *Spirits and Demons at Work: Alcohol and Other Drugs on the Job*. Ithaca: New York State School of Industrial and Labor Relations, Cornell University.

Williams, R. L. 1975. "The evaluation of Occupational Health Services, Inc., Oakland, California." Unpublished manuscript.

Williams, R. L., and D. Lindley. 1975. "A method to determine on-the-job production impairment." Unpublished manuscript.

Williams, R. L., and G. H. Moffat, eds. 1975. *Occupational Alcoholism Programs*. Springfield, Ill.: Charles C Thomas.

Williams, R. L., and R. Temer. 1975. "Evaluation—a model: The evaluation of occupational programming: What it is, what it isn't, and how to do it!'' Paper presented at the International ALMACA Meeting, Atlanta, Ga.

Winslow, W. W., K. Hayes, L. Prentice, W. E. Powles, W. Seeman, and W. D. Ross. 1966. ''Some economic estimates of job disruption from an industrial mental health project.'' *Archives of Environmental Health* 13:213–19.

Wrich, J. T. 1974. *The Employee Assistance Program.* Center City, Minn. Hazelden.

PART III

NINE / The Development of a Successful Alcoholism Treatment Facility

CARL J. SCHRAMM

In 1972, the United States Department of Labor underwrote a study proposed by the Johns Hopkins University School of Hygiene and Public Health to develop basic research on the labor-force behavior of alcoholic workers. In order to assemble a population of alcoholic workers of sufficient size for the study, the Employee Health Program (EHP), a single-situs treatment facility to which several Baltimore companies and unions would refer problem-drinking workers for treatment, was established. The decision to operate a clinic was made for reasons beyond the goals of research, however. By offering a single set of referral, counseling, and treatment services that could be shared by a number of employers and unions, EHP sought to test a new concept in reaching and rehabilitating problem drinkers at the work place.

A major form of federal support for company-based treatment efforts had been the funding of demonstration projects designed to explore the feasibility of alternative models for reaching employed problem drinkers. The basic emphasis of most of these projects had been for the employer and/or union to assume the major responsibility for the program after the demonstration phase. Similarly, a condition of the grant establishing EHP was that the clinic strive for self-sufficiency during the three years of funding. Essentially, the consortium, or multi-employer approach, exemplified by EHP was a demonstration project to determine whether a single set of referral, counseling, and treatment services shared by several employers and unions was a workable treatment model. Thus, takeover of the clinic by participating employers and/or unions after expiration of federal funding would serve as proof of both the need for and the acceptability of the multiparty concept. The decision to operate EHP as an outpatient facility, however, was seen as one possible obstacle to its prospects for self-sufficiency

---

The author wishes to acknowledge grant 21-24-73-23 from the United States Department of Labor, Employment and Training Administration, which provided funds for the research reported here.

because, at the time of EHP's inception, insurance coverage for outpatient treatment for alcoholism was virtually nonexistent.

Therefore, the major goals of the demonstration project were first to determine whether such a single-situs concept could be made operational and, second, whether it could become self-sustaining. During the 29 months from the opening of the clinic in June 1973 until the expiration of federal funding on 31 October 1975, the project accomplished both tasks. EHP had emerged as an autonomous, community-owned treatment program with ties extending far beyond its original member firms and unions. As an organization faced with the complexities of coordinating the efforts and interests of multiple parties, in addition to those inherent in launching a new clinical effort, EHP offers experiences that encompass a broad range of issues in the field of industrial alcoholism. Following a brief description of the organizational structure and goals of EHP, this chapter describes, in broad, chronologic form, the problems encountered by EHP in developing a new treatment concept and the solutions devised to overcome them.

STRUCTURE AND FUNCTIONS

Organization and Staff

The day-to-day management and locus of decision-making within EHP fell to the project's executive committee. The committee was responsible to the university's central administration, which in turn was the contracting party to the Department of Labor. The executive committee was composed of the principal investigator, the director of clinic treatment (the clinic's head counselor), the director of clinic administration (the clinic's business officer), and the director of research. Also joining the executive committee on an irregular basis was the clinic's psychiatrist. The executive committee met weekly to oversee the project's activities.

The purpose of the advisory board—composed of representatives of the participating managements and unions, as well as several members of the Baltimore alcoholism community—was to advise the executive committee and to consider policies for stabilizing and continuing the program after the demonstration phase. Over the course of the two years, the advisory relationship changed considerably. In the beginning, the executive committee had to devise agendas for the advisory board, as well as specify its functions. Later, the board took its own initiative, and the executive committee became subordinated to it in many areas, including personnel, the admission of new employers to the programs, and the question of clinic ownership after university withdrawal.

In direct-line authority under the executive committee were the Baltimore Area Council on Alcoholism (BACA), the Metropolitan Baltimore Council of AFL-CIO Unions, the clinic staff, and the research personnel. BACA was under contract to the executive committee to develop in-service training programs for personnel in the participating industries and to act as liaison with management representatives of member employers. The Council of AFL-CIO unions established liaison with participating unions.

Essentially, four types of personnel were employed by the project: physicians, counselors, liaison officers, and clerk-secretaries. As of the summer of 1975, three part-time physicians attended the program, with each supplying about four hours per week.

By far the most important personnel were the counselors. The project attempted to keep the case load of each at or below 35. Because new referrals require extra attention, it was an operating rule that in any one month a counselor would handle no more than five new cases. Given the growing active case load, the number of counselors grew from two to five by the end of the second year. A number of criteria were used in selecting counselors. First, since black patients formed a large percentage of the case load, it became important to have several black counselors with whom patients could develop a special relationship. While at no time were patients assigned to counselors on the basis of race, the presence of black counselors in the clinic and in the conduct of group therapy sessions proved reassuring to black patients. A second criterion was to maintain a mix of women and men on the counseling staff. Female counselors proved to be very effective, especially in working with black male patients. Two female counselors worked in the clinic throughout the second year of operation. Finally, the counseling staff always included at least one recovered alcoholic who was a member of Alcoholics Anonymous. The presence of a recovered alcoholic served as a constant object lesson to patients that recovery was possible.

Since employers and unions would need both stimulation and support in their efforts to refer alcoholic employees to the clinic, the project appointed liaison personnel to provide educational and training services as well as to oversee the interaction of participating employers and unions with the project. The principal criteria used in selecting liaison personnel were their potential acceptability to participating managements and unions and a thoroughgoing understanding of alcoholism as a problem in the work force.

Secretarial needs were substantial because of the detailed records kept on each patient and the volume of telephone calls and correspondence required to keep track of referred patients. The program employed two secretaries and a receptionist at the close of the second year of clinic operation.

The Complex of Goals, Tasks, and Assessors

Although EHP was a relatively small effort (at no time did it employ more than 15 persons), its widely divergent program goals and tasks suggest that it be considered a complex organization. The theorists of organizational science pose a dichotomous model of organizations relative to the degree of integration of their tasks. As will be seen shortly, the tasks of EHP were highly resistent to integration and thus presented greater management problems than those facing a simple organization.[1] The project attempted both a demonstration and a research mission, which by nature involve incompatible goals and tasks. Research is best accomplished in stable settings, while a demonstration effort requires a fluid, dynamic, and adventurous organizational concept. The problem is compounded when the objective of research is to evaluate demonstration goals; the research effort will naturally press for organizational stability in the short run, while the demonstration concerns willl press for change.

Within the demonstration part of the project itself—i.e., the clinic effort—were several subgoals and tasks which also stood in partial opposition to each other. The first such goal was program growth. This involved the substantial task of promoting active and enthusiastic cooperation between labor and management participants to generate a sufficient case load to justify the project's existence. A second goal was cost constraint. Despite the need for an all-out expenditure on stimulating patient referrals, resources had to be kept in reserve in the event that radically different methods of patient recruitment might be required. Moreover, the goals of high-quality patient care involved a high level of physician attention, which was very costly to purchase. Another goal was unobtrusive entrance into the community and the maintenance of a low organizational profile. This goal conflicted with efforts to promote program growth, since greater publicity would be likely to advance the referral effort. Finally, a major goal was eventual financial self-sustenance for the program and its reorganization as an on-going community resource. Here, the task was to balance the interests of both unions and employers as potential supporters of the clinic after university withdrawal,

1. The notion of simple and complex organizations is discussed in Thompson 1967. The criterion of organizational complexity accepted in this chapter is the degree of integration possible among all the goals and tasks assumed by an organization. By this standard, organizations such as small retail outlets, manufacturing concerns, and savings and loan associations permitting a high degree of integration are simple organizations.

while maintaining their good will and cooperation in the day-to-day operations of the program. Acting together, these often conflicting goals and tasks rendered management of the project immensely difficult.

In addition to the combination of diverging goals and tasks, the assessment environment in which the project operated was also characteristic of a complex organization. The assessment environment is that collectivity of interests and individuals (''significant others'') which must be satisfied by the organization's performance if the organization is to survive and grow in the future.[2] Six parties made up the assessment environment of EHP: (1) the two government agencies which funded the project; (2) participating employers, who controlled and provided the bulk of referrals and who held the promise for future financial backing; (3) participating unions, who also had to be pleased with clinic operations and who also held the promise of future funding; (4) the Joint Comission on Accreditation, which alone could provide external legitimacy to EHP; (5) the insurance carrier promising to be a potential source of the future financial viability of the program; and, to a lesser extent, (6) the medical and alcoholism ''establishments'' in the community, which held the power to endorse or repudiate the EHP effort.

In the face of this multiplicity of assessors, the project had to establish a priority of interests to recognize and serve. Throughout most of the project's experience, the Department of Labor was its preeminent assessor by force of its role as exclusive funder. However, as in any situation in which a number of persons or groups have established themselves as having an interest in the organization and as being potential providers for its future support, the project was forced to establish secondary and tertiary priorities among competing assessors. This involved creating a number of fictions for various assessors regarding their importance to the project. One illustration was the portrayal of the importance of integration with a specific halfway house as a means of reducing community resistance. Although necessary in keeping all assessors satisfied, such fictions could become confusing, and periodically, project management would have to evaluate the importance of assessors' demands and needs and decide in what order of priority they should be met.

A final complexity of the assessment environment was the changing priority of assessors over time. While the priorities of the Department of Labor were preeminent throughout the first two years, secondary priorities became more dynamic

2. For a discussion of ''significant others'' in the life of an organization attempting to demonstrate its ''fitness for the future,'' see Thompson 1967 and Schramm 1975.

during the summer of 1975, when, as will be seen below, the Community Service Agency (CSA) promised to become the long-term sponsor of the project.

In sum, as will become clear in the following description of the operating history of the project, the management and administration of EHP was made particularly complex by the conflicting nature of its goals and tasks and by the multitude of its assessors and their changing status over time. In the two years of the demonstration phase, EHP can be seen as having passed through three stages: (1) initiation; (2) reorganization, consolidation, and growth; and (3) insuring self-sustenance. At each stage, the project faced a different series of obstacles and challenges. By examining in detail several of the problems and solutions as they emerged, the balance of this chapter presents EHP experiences which should be of interest to those hoping to start similar social action programs.

INITIATING A NEW TREATMENT FACILITY

Any new health-care facility faces two immediate tasks: gaining acceptance by the community as providing an acceptable level of services, and establishing a clientele. Although EHP was identified with a respected medical institution (Johns Hopkins) and had a prearranged clientele, the first year of clinic operation was a struggle to fulfill both tasks.

The Problem of Community Resistance

The project's planners had anticipated that EHP would meet with a certain degree of community resistance as it sought to gain acceptance in a metropolitan area which already had eight outpatient, inpatient, and part-way residential programs devoted exclusively to the treatment of alcoholics. Organizational theory suggested that a new program, particularly one which projected a high-level professional image and which established an "exclusive" target catchment population, would be seen as a threat to existing programs and an implied criticism of the level of services that they provided. Moreover, the communality among persons working in the field of alcoholism treatment—a phenomenon that Trice and Roman (1972) refer to as the "alcoholism industry"—was recognized by the project's planners. Finally, the Baltimore alcoholism treatment community has always appeared to be suspicious of treatment efforts not in the tradition of Alcoholics Anonymous. EHP, with its staff of physicians, psychiatrists, counselors, and liaison personnel, was certain to contrast with that tradition.

In anticipation of these problems the project planners devised three strategies to minimize community resistance to EHP. The first was to integrate a highly visible part of the established alcoholism community into the project by turning over the labor and management liaison activities to the Baltimore Area Council on Alcoholism. The second was to develop and structure a community advisory board that would have actual decision-making power and that would eventually take an ownership interest in the project. By asking a number of the most visible leaders of the alcoholism establishment to serve on the board, a direct channel would be opened for communicating the project's views on all issues to the persons who ultimately could decide the future of the project, namely, those who controlled referrals. The third strategy was to insure that the counseling staff of the project always included at least one person who was a member of Alcoholics Anonymous (AA). While having no formal structure, AA provides a common experience of such impact that its members share in a social network of great strength. Establishing the credibility of the program with this network was important because many of the counselors working in other community agencies and programs were former alcoholics who had recovered with the help of AA. Additionally, several participating employers and unions had AA members serving as full- or part-time alcoholism counselors or had an employee known to be a former alcoholic whom they could call upon to help other alcoholic workers.

Despite these attempts to ease the project into the community, resistance began to mount shortly after the program became operational and persisted throughout the first six months. The resistance took several forms, including the circulation of stories portraying the research interests of the project as involving experimental medical and psychiatric treatment, as well as an increased interest in EHP employers by other alcoholism programs, who reminded them that they could send problem workers to longer-established treatment facilities.

Because of this unanticipated level of resistance, the project began to establish communications with the other treatment facilities and programs in an attempt to dispel their fears and to suggest possible avenues for cooperation. For example, the project worked out arrangements with residential programs to refer to them EHP patients needing inpatient care. Those facilities, funded on the basis of patient volume, were allowed to count both the patients they referred to EHP and the EHP patients sent to them. In one case, negotiations were made for EHP to integrate with one treatment center as its outpatient facility, though the linkage was never effected because of the physical remoteness of that center.

The problem posed by community resistance began to ebb about the sixth month of clinic operations, at which time overtures were made to the program to join the local alcoholism establishment. The author is convinced, however, that the most important factor in this change of attitude was the low rate of patients referred to EHP during the first six months. Thus, only when programs became reassured that EHP did not decrease demand for other services was it welcomed as a member of the existing treatment community.

The Problem of Generating Patient Load

The program was originally funded through a joint mechanism bringing together three years of support from both the National Institute on Alcohol Abuse and Alcoholism (NIAAA) and the U. S. Department of Labor. Since its founding in 1971, NIAAA has shifted between two approaches regarding the proper treatment of industrial alcoholism. The EHP project was conceived and funded during a time when NIAAA was stressing programs dealing exclusively with alcoholism, but during the summer of 1973, institute policy was rapidly shifting towards broad-brush approaches.[3] Since NIAAA was also faced with budgetary cut-backs, its new priorities, coupled with an internal estimate of EHP's chance for survival, led to the institute's withdrawal of support from the project in September 1973. The Department of Labor was then faced with the decision of whether to nearly triple its original funding commitment to insure the continuation of the project. An evaluation of the clinical operation was begun, and it soon focused on the poor rate of referrals to the clinic.

Though original projections had called for an annual load of 250 patients, there had been only 52 referrals to the clinic during the initial six months. In part, the slow rate of referrals was due to factors largely beyond the control of the project—community resistance and the fact that the clinic had opened in June (July and August are traditionally slow months for referrals in all medical programs). Therefore, the outcome of the Labor Department's evaluation was a decision to continue funding for a six-month trial period to determine whether referrals could be increased to a rate which would produce a large enough population to meet the research goals of the project.

To accomplish this, the number of participating employers was expanded from eight to twelve, thus increasing the work force at risk from 89,000 to 134,000. In addition, one labor liaison and one management liaison were added to the staff, effectively doubling referral-stimulating capacities. As a result of these steps, the

3. The broad-brush approach argues that potential labeling and stigmatization are the most significant barriers to effectively getting alcoholism treatment to industrial populations and, thus, any therapeutic efforts should be organized as part of a larger and presumably less threatening "troubled employees" effort which would deal with a host of psychopathologies presented by workers. The reverse position is that advocating programs designed to deal exclusively with alcoholic workers. The broad-brush versus exclusively alcoholism debate is discussed by Roman and Trice (1976).

second six months saw an increase of 79 new patients referred to the clinic. Satisfied with the project's ability to generate cases, in March 1974, the Labor Department decided to provide an additional 18 months of funding.

REORGANIZATION, CONSOLIDATION, AND GROWTH

The clinic was able to survive the crisis raised by the slow rate of referrals during the first year of clinic operation, but not without serious disruptions. Since the treatment staff had been developed to handle a growing case load of about 20 new patients a month, staff members were becoming bored and anxious in the face of a seemingly small demand for their services. This, coupled with uncertainty over future funding, prompted staff members to investigate other employment prospects. The net result was that the entire counseling staff had to be replaced in the last months of the first year. Thus, the second year of clinic operation began with a new staff and, as will be seen below, a new administration.

Issues in Clinic Administration

The crisis surrounding the slow rate of patient referrals precipitated a reevaluation of all aspects of clinic operation, including its administration. Alcoholism treatment programs can be broadly divided into those which operate on a medical model and those which operate on a social service model. Programs following the medical model have a high degree of physician input and operate on the assumption of physical illness; patients enter treatment by referral and are individually diagnosed, treated, and released. In the social service model, the major professional input is from counselors and social workers, entrance is gained through a default process (as in public inebriate programs, in which the alcoholic has no other place to go), and treatment consists of adjusting the individual's environment as well as counseling him. Progress through treatment is not always clear, and a discrete discharge point is seldom reached. While EHP had elements of both the medical and social service models, it most clearly resembled the medical model. Treatment was always under the supervision of physicians and was based on a disease concept of alcoholism. EHP patients were referred by a fixed number of employers or unions, and the treatment process was viewed as close-ended.

Consistent with its adherence to a medical model, the project employed a physician on a full-time basis to oversee the treatment of patients and the organization of the clinic. This proved to be a very costly deployment of physician hours because there was an actual demand for only 10 to 15 hours of medical care per week, but at least 30 hours were required for administrative chores. Moreover, the status of physicians in a broader societal context makes it particularly difficult to deal with them as employees. At several key points, the executive committee had problems in getting the physician-director conform to its policies and procedures. Consequently, at the end of the first year, the physician-director was replaced by a full-time administrator and a counselor-director, and part-time physicians were recruited from among community-based general practitioners and medical residents in nearby hospitals.

TABLE 9.1 NEW REFERRALS AND CLINICAL VISITS BY MONTH

Month	*Referrals*	*Cumulative Total*	*Clinic Revisits**	*Cumulative Total*
June 1973	3		11	
July	9	12	35	46
August	4	16	42	88
September	8	24	64	152
October	15	39	83	235
November	13	52	92	327
December	11	63	99	426
January 1974	19	82	121	547
February	14	96	136	683
March	12	108	141	824
April	12	120	152	976
May	11	131	137	1,113
June	15	146	123†	1,236
July	15	161	215	1,451
August	25	186	301	1,752
September	17	203	347	2,099
October	18	221	427	2,526
November	24	245	363	2,889
December	22	267	382	3,271
January 1975	15	282	409	3,680
February	17	299	331	4,011
March	14	313	360	4,371
April	17	330	376	4,387
May	23	353	429	4,816
June	16	369	573	5,389
July	22	391	523	5,912

*Includes all visits less new visits.

†This low reflected the inevitable disruption in patient care which occurred as a result of the complete changeover in counseling staff.

Accessibility of Treatment

Another issue that emerged during EHP's period of self-scrutiny was the geographic location of the clinic. Because of concerns for patients' safety, attractive surroundings, and access to the city's high-speed beltway, the clinic was located in a professional building in a suburban neighborhood north of the city. After the clinic had been operating for several months, however, it became apparent that the persons making referrals were reluctant to offer the long trip to the clinic as the only treatment option and that some workers who were referred dropped out rather than make the trip on a periodic basis. Consequently, a survey of EHP patients' traveling experiences was conducted, and it was found that the bulk of the patient population lived along an east-west axis in the community far from the clinic. The survey also uncovered the fact that many workers felt uneasy about the suburban location itself. To a person who had spent the majority of his life in a lower-income, predominantly black neighborhood, the clinic represented a threatening experience.

The staff began to examine alternative sites closer to the center of the city, and a new site was chosen that was convenient both to the residences and places of employment of the majority of patients. The decision to relocate was immediately vindicated in both referral and revisit rates. Table 9.1 shows the response in revisits after moving the clinic in early October 1974.

Routinization of the Referral Mechanism

In many respects increase in patient load is the best measure of clinic growth. By the end of the second year the ratio of active cases to referrals, which had been 0.49 at the end of the first 12 months, decreased to 0.32 because of the discharge of patients seen during the first year and the stabilization of new referrals at about 20 per month during the second.

It had been an operating hypothesis of the project's management that once the program was firmly established in the community, new referrals would be made without stimulation. Consequently, during the third six-month period, the project's liaison activity was cut back to one person each in management and labor. Evidence that the hypothesis was correct came in the first six months of 1975, when the impact of a reduction in liaison activity should have been felt. As Table 9.1 shows, both clinic referral and revisit rates continued to increase. In June, the management liaison position was cut back to a half-time job, and the labor liaison activity was halted altogether.

PROMOTING FINANCIAL SELF-SUFFICIENCY

From the outset of the project one goal dominated all others—the eventual transformation of the clinic from a federally financed and university-operated demonstration into a financially independent, community-owned treatment resource. In working toward this goal the project's management realized that it had to make the program as attractive as possible to participating employers and unions in two areas—effective treatment of referred patients and potential financial self-sufficiency.

It was easier to influence clients' perceptions about treatment, for two reasons. First, the clinic was in a position to affect the outcomes of patient treatment but had no power to make decisions about future financing since all of the resources lay in the hands of employers, unions, and health insurance underwriters. Second, whereas there were few external criteria that participating managements and unions could use to measure the quality of treatment, the project had to offer objective evidence that EHP could be economically self-sustaining at the end of grant funding. Therefore, the most critical area of strategy for project management in ensuring continuation of the clinic was to secure a long-term source of income to meet future operating costs.

The Funding Options

Three major avenues of future funding for the clinic were under consideration from the time of initial project planning: fee-for-service payment, underwriting by the participating parties, and third-part reimbursement.

The fee-for-service method presumed either that patients referred to the clinic would pay cash for services rendered and be reimbursed by the employer, or that employers would send payment directly to the clinic for treatment received by their employees. A disadvantage of the fee-for-service method was that most employers are not equipped to pay health-care bills directly because of the role played by third-party carriers. An employer reimbursement scheme would have involved establishing a new set of procedures and policies in the employers' purchasing departments.

The second funding option was financing via a subscription mechanism through which participating employers and unions would underwrite all the costs of clinic operations. This concept would have permitted greater latitude in managing the clinic than the fee-for-service option, since, with all costs underwritten, clinic growth could be controlled by actual demand for services rather than by the need to maintain large patient loads to maximize fee-for-service revenues. The problems associated with this type of financing were primarily equity concerns among the parties. While some employers might have been willing to make a fixed gift to the project, others argued for a cost-sharing scheme, pro-rated to the employer's use of the clinic; still others doubted whether they could contribute at all.

The third option was a third-party payment mechanism whereby the employer's health-care insurer or a union welfare fund would reimburse the clinic for all services actually rendered to referred workers. This option was attractive for many reasons. Foremost was that since third-party reimbursement is the most widely accepted and understood means of health-care policy, the problem of finding an acceptable or common third-party payer never arose. Additionally, insurance companies had already established a modality for arranging payment and would provide a system of uniform rates acceptable to all parties. Finally, the employer's contribution to the clinic would be relatively painless under such a plan. The health carrier would add an across-the-board premium onto the employers' policies that would be inconsequential relative to the total premiums paid for all health and surgical coverage.

While the health-care insurer option appeared to be the most attractive, there were many hurdles to be crossed before it could be implemented. First, only one or two health insurance carriers in the United States offered limited outpatient alcoholism benefits on an experimental basis. Thus, the participating employers were unable to purchase an existing benefit package in Maryland. Second, the employers were hesitant about purchasing such benefits since the concept of outpatient treatment paid for by the employer was untested in Baltimore and only experimented with elsewhere. Third, before an underwriter would reimburse, the clinic would have to be certified as meeting standards, but there was no mechanism for accrediting outpatient alcoholism facilities. Finally, even if health carriers were to offer a plan for outpatient alcoholism treatment benefits, it would have to be approved by the state insurance commission.

The Development of Third-Party Reimbursement

Because each of the three systems held some appeal and because no single system became the clear choice for future financing of the project, all three options had to be pursued throughout the first 18 months of the project's existence. But early in 1974, through its appointee to the project's advisory board, Blue Cross of Maryland began a preliminary inquiry into the costs of operating EHP and of delivering outpatient alcoholism benefits. Changing Blue Cross's initial interest in outpatient alcoholism treatment into an actual source of funding was a complex and prolonged process which should be of interest to those who would like to replicate the EHP experience.

The first phase was to develop Blue Cross's commitment to the concept of underwriting outpatient alcoholism services. This task was facilitated in the case of Maryland Blue Cross by its already high degree of interest in the general problem of alcoholism. Maryland Blue Cross had been the first such carrier in the nation to reimburse inpatient care for alcoholics. Through the efforts of both labor and management members of the advisory board and of Blue Cross's appointee to the board, who actively communicated to his superiors the growing consumer interest in outpatient coverage, Blue Cross was alerted to the developing need for a benefit package that would provide to its subscribers outpatient services of the kind offered by EHP. Moreover, several union leaders met with the senior account executives of Maryland Blue Cross and indicated that they were committed to negotiate alcoholism treatment benefits at the next round of contract renewals, covering some 30,000 to 50,000 employees. They requested that Blue Cross prepare rates which could be used in collective bargaining. Thus, EHP contributed to the development of outpatient coverage by presenting persons (unions) ready to purchase services.

Achieving Accreditation

As part of the process of preparing for Blue Cross reimbursement, the clinic had to be formally recognized as providing satisfactory and acceptable care by satisfying the requirements that the health professionals providing the services be licensed practitioners and that the delivery institution be accredited by a recognized body of health-care providers. Since outpatient alcoholism programs are relative newcomers among health-care delivery institutions, at the beginning of the project there was no existing group responsible for certifying such programs. The steps toward solving this problem began in the fall of 1974, when the Joint Commission on Hospital Accreditation (JCHA) announced that it would develop criteria for outpatient alcoholism programs and facilities to be tested on a trial basis in Maryland as well as in two other states. Upon this announcement, EHP immediately applied to JCHA for an accreditation evaluation. In March 1975, a two-man team was sent from Chicago to evaluate EHP in terms of 200 clinical and administrative criteria. The examiners cited the project as being far above the expectations developed by the commission for outpatient alcoholism programs. EHP received a two-year accreditation certificate and was chosen by JCHA as an unofficial model program.

The EHP Fee Schedule

For the clinic, the most important task involved in developing the third-party payer mechanism was to create a schedule of fees which would be reimbursed by Blue Cross. Since EHP was the only outpatient clinic in the state to work with Blue Cross in developing program benefits, its estimates would have an obvious impact on programs to follow. For this reason, and because the clinic would be

TABLE 9.2 THE EMPLOYEE HEALTH PROGRAM PATIENT FEE SCHEDULE

Procedure	*Fee**	*Total*
First 30 Days		
Treatment plan preparation		
2 initial interviews	$35	$ 70
1 physical examination	40	40
1 psychiatric examination	40	40
1 physical follow-up	15	15
1 staff-patient conference	25	25
1 laboratory test (blood-urine)	25	25
Post-treatment plan counseling		
5 individual therapy visits	25	125
3 group therapy visits	15	45
Subsequent Visits†		
Individual therapy visits	25	500
Group therapy visits	15	300
		$1185

*The fees were determined by prorating actual expenses of the several clinical activities across all patients and allowing for a normal period of time in treatment. In the case of physical and psychiatric examinations, the fees represent actual payments to the physicians plus an overhead allowance. Laboratory fees are charged without clinic overhead since they are subcontracted to a laboratory which can bill Blue Cross directly. The fees of $25.00 for individual counseling and $15.00 for group therapy reflect true costs plus overhead. These figures were determined by taking all costs less physician and laboratory expenses and dividing by the number of individual and group visits for the six-month period 1 January through 30 June 1975.

†While the number of individual and group visits after the first 30 days may vary, the typical patient would require about 20 individual therapy visits and 20 group therapy sessions.

forced to maintain itself on its reimbursed fees, great care and study went into preparing the schedule (Table 9.2).

Eventually, Blue Cross developed three outpatient alcoholism plans which offered employers and other subscribers a range of benefits, with per-individual premiums of $0.08 per month for the least comprehensive and $0.20 for the most comprehensive plan. In September 1975, the State Insurance Commission gave Blue Cross approval to market all three plans for outpatient treatment. On October 1, Blue Cross began wide-scale publicity aimed at the community at large, with specific promotional efforts directed to its 17,000 employer subscribers.

FUTURE OWNERSHIP AND CONTROL OF EHP

During the spring of 1975, the project's advisory board appointed a subcommittee to consider the question of ownership of the clinic after the university's withdrawal. The subcommittee considered three principal options. The first was a nonprofit community corporation managed by the project's advisory board. This option would have moved the clinic into a fee-for-service financial structure, preserving the staffing pattern that had evolved during the first two years. The second was a nonprofit community corporation which would seek continuing institutional support for its major financing and would contract for services with a separate corporation composed of the project's treatment staff. The third option was to turn the project over *in toto* to one of the two groups interested in operating it—the Metropolitan Baltimore AFL-CIO or the Baltimore Area Council on Alcoholism.

Almost from the start, the committee was destined to choose the third option. The most compelling reason was that such an arrangement would provide for immediate financial sponsorship. Moreover, both BACA and the AFL-CIO displayed enthusiasm, while there was an apparent lack of sponsorship for the other two options. The emergence of BACA and AFL-CIO interest in taking over EHP provides an interesting insight into the project's impact on the community. Throughout the first year of clinic operation, BACA had been increasingly uncomfortable with the role organized labor played in the project, a concern stemming mainly from its previous favorable experiences with management interest in alcoholism. Additionally, some management representatives to the advisory board felt a need to form a loose confederation or caucus to counter the natural bond that joined the union representatives from the onset. Although the management caucus seemed to have BACA influence in its bid for project ownership, it never emerged as a controlling force on the advisory board. Management representatives were never empowered by their superiors to commit employer resources; thus, even though the caucus gave the appearance of a cohesive management viewpoint or interest, it could not act decisively.

The bid by the Baltimore AFL-CIO was grounded in circumstances considerably beyond the scope of the project. During recent years, the organized labor movement has expressed growing concern over its ability to stimulate and influence existing public and private social welfare agencies, voluntary community treatment facilities (e.g., neighborhood health centers), and major hospitals to deliver high-quality care to its members. As a result, the AFL-CIO had decided to organize a number of such activities under a union aegis called the Community Service Agency (CSA). CSA was incorporated in early 1975 and began to plan various projects. Since the director of CSA was also a member of the advisory board of EHP and one of the initiators of the EHP experiment, it was only natural that CSA set out to take on the project as its first activity. The board's attraction to this option was that CSA proposed to leave the EHP plan virtually intact and would continue the advisory board in its present mix of labor and management. The BACA plan, on the other hand, implied to union leaders a change in operating goals—i.e., making the project somehow more responsive to management. The AFL-CIO plan was endorsed by the advisory board in July 1975 and plans for the university's divestiture on behalf of CSA were put into effect.

In retrospect, the CSA plan was bound to win out over BACA's bid for a number of reasons. First, the AFL-CIO pledged itself to full financial support of the project at the advisory board meeting in July. BACA was in no position to make a similar guarantee. Second, the management caucus was not displeased in any discernible way with how the program was being operated and, thus, any attempt to form the management representatives into an effective dissident group would be likely to fail. Third, the union representatives had repeatedly displayed both unquestionable loyalty to the program and genuine fairness in all issues debated by advisory council. A spirit of good faith and trust linked the union members of the council, who had seen the project through hard times and had been jointly pleased with the project's emerging predominence. Finally, the AFL-CIO proposal defused any management objection by providing for a continuing role for management representatives in the policy-making board of EHP.

As the project closed its second year of operation, its future looked both secure and bright. It would be taken over by the community and was enjoying both a local and national reputation for excellent treatment. Everything proceeded as planned and on October 31, the university turned control of the project over to CSA.

EHP continued to operate under the aegis of CSA until fall, 1976, when insufficient funds forced the clinic to close. Despite the success of the project in laying the groundwork for long-term financing (through development of the Blue Cross reimbursement coverage) there were insufficient short-term funds to support clinic activities until such time as the reimbursement mechanism could become capable of supporting total operating costs. The Blue Cross outpatient package was not marketed until October, 1975, and although the benefits have attracted many subscribers, extension of coverage to a sufficient number of workers to sustain the clinic did not occur soon enough. Many EHP employers had been in fixed contracts with Blue Cross and could not purchase the new services until their present contracts had expired and new ones could be negotiated. It is likely that, had the clinic been able to continue for about two years under CSA management, all referred patients would have been covered by the Blue Cross plans of their employers. Government funds remaining after the demonstration phase were sufficient to operate the clinic only for about six months. After that period, the AFL–CIO paid for the clinic out of its own reserves. No other support was forthcoming either from government or from the participating employers. Unable to continue providing all of the interim funding needed, the CSA had to close the clinic, and EHP patients were then shifted over to the alcoholism program of The Johns Hopkins Hospital.

REFERENCES

Roman, P. M., and H. M. Trice. 1976. "Alcohol abuse and work organizations." In B. Kissen and H. Begleiter, eds., *The Biology of Alcoholism,* vol. 4, pp. 445–517. New York: Plenum Press.

Schramm, C. J. 1975. "Thompson's assessment of organizations: Universities and the AAUP salary grades." *Administrative Science Quarterly* 20:87–96.

Thompson, J. 1967. *Organizations in Action.* New York: McGraw-Hill.

Trice, H. M., and P. M. Roman. 1972. *Spirits and Demons at Work: Alcohol and Other Drugs on the Job.* Ithaca: New York State School of Industrial and Labor Relations, Cornell University.

TEN / Social Stability, Work Force Behavior, and Job Satisfaction of Alcoholic and Nonalcoholic Blue-Collar Workers

JANET ARCHER

From June 1973 to October 1975 The Johns Hopkins University operated an outpatient alcoholism clinic for workers referred for treatment by 12 employers and unions in Metropolitan Baltimore. Known as the Employee Health Program (EHP), the facility served both as a demonstration of the feasibility of a single-situs treatment clinic for use by multiple employers and unions, as well as a mechanism for assembling a study population for research. The major goals of the research component of the project were to develop basic data on the work force characteristics of alcoholics and to assess the efficacy of therapeutic intervention in improving their labor force participation.

Previous research, reviewed in Chapter 1 of this volume, has yielded a small body of basic knowledge on the characteristics of employed problem drinkers,[1] as well as many untested suggestions. It is generally agreed that although problem-drinking workers remain in the labor force while in the early and middle stages of their affliction, and tend to have many years of service with their employers, little is known of the factors that may distinguish them from their non-problem-drinking counterparts in the work force. A number of studies have hypothesized a link between alcohol misuse and employment-related stresses, such as dissatisfaction with job content, working conditions, and span of control (O'Toole 1973). If such a link exists, it should be reflected in greater job dissatisfaction among alcoholics than nonalcoholics when both are exposed to similar work situations.

In order to explore the characteristics and attitudes that might differentiate

1. The terms *alcoholic* and *problem drinker* are used interchangeably in this paper. The controversy surrounding the issue of terminology is discussed in Chapter 1 of this book.

alcoholic from nonalcoholic workers, the EHP project assembled a comparison group of workers drawn from the work forces of the same employers from which the study population was referred. This article will report some differences and similarities that emerged from a comparison of both groups of workers with respect to social stability, work behavior, and job and life satisfactions.

The population of alcoholic workers described here consists only of those workers who were identified as alcoholic and referred for treatment and is not a representative sample of alcoholics in the referring companies' labor forces. As will be seen below, the EHP study population consisted primarily of blue-collar workers employed in manufacturing companies. While this population does not serve as a basis for making generalizations about the characteristics of employed alcoholics, it does afford us the opportunity to examine job satisfaction among a category of workers who are most likely to experience the employment-related dissatisfactions thought to promote heavy use of alcohol as a coping device. Additionally, although our data on the social and work force characteristics of the study population should be viewed as primarily descriptive, they can be compared with findings on alcoholic workers from other treatment populations. Moreover, when presented along with similar data for a comparison group of nonproblem drinkers, they do suggest a need to reconsider a number of our conceptions of the correlates of alcohol misuse by workers.

THE STUDY AND COMPARISON POPULATIONS

The findings on alcoholic workers reported in this chapter consist primarily of data obtained from a questionnaire administered to each study worker during the first two weeks of his interface with the clinic. The study population was restricted to the first patients seen at the clinic during the two-year demonstration in order to allow a sufficient time interval between intake and review to assess the impact of treatment. Of the 219 patients who answered questionnaires, only 13 were women, largely because the majority of referrals were made by manufacturing companies with predominantly male work forces. Because there were so few women, the study population was restricted to the 206 male referrals.

The comparison group consisted of 100 male workers employed by the twelve referring companies. Because the participating companies were reluctant to supply the project with the names and addresses of their work forces, the comparison group was obtained using telephone listings from Baltimore-area neighborhoods. Using an abbreviated version of the intake questionnaire, we conducted telephone interviews, matching respondents with study workers on age, race, and

TABLE 10.1 PERCENTAGE DISTRIBUTION OF DRINKING TYPES FOR THE COMPARISON GROUP AND ADP SURVEY OPERATIVES

Drinking Type	*Comparison Group*	*ADP Survey Male Operatives**
Abstainers	20	27
Infrequent drinkers	15	12
Light and moderate drinkers	38	35
Heavy drinkers	27	26
	100	100
Percentage of all drinkers who are heavy drinkers	34%	36%

*The modal occupation of comparison workers

occupation. An equivalent breakdown by race was obtained. The groups proved to be very similar with respect to income, education, and state of birth. Comparison workers had a median age four years older than the study population, and with the exception of service workers (of whom there were none in the comparison group) the occupational distribution was comparable.

In order to establish that the comparison group was, in fact, a sample of nonalcoholic, non-problem-drinking workers, the responses of this group to questions on drinking behavior were examined using criteria set down by Cahalan et al. (1969) in their survey of normal American drinking practices (ADP). The comparison workers were classified as shown in Table 10.1. Given the similarity between the percentage distributions for the comparison and the ADP workers, it is reasonable to conclude that the drinking behavior of the comparison group was characteristic of that of a normal population of industrial workers. Only two comparison workers reported having had any problems connected with alcohol consumption in the month preceding the interview, and none reported having received treatment for alcoholism at any time in the past.

CHARACTERISTICS OF THE EHP STUDY POPULATION AT INTAKE

Following a description of the drinking histories reported by EHP referrals, this section will present selected demographic and socioeconomic characteristics of the 206 male workers comprising the study population. The section will conclude by contrasting the study and comparison workers with respect to social stability.

Drinking History and Attitudes toward Referral and Treatment

As a rule, workers are not referred to industrial alcoholism programs for treatment until their problem has progressed to the middle or late stages of alcoholism (Trice 1965). Because EHP served as the first alcoholism identification and referral program for most of the participating employers, it is not surprising that the majority of the study population were found to have had a long history of heavy drinking and of problems associated with excessive consumption of alcohol.

Sixty-five percent of the study population reported that they had been drinking heavily for ten or more years prior to coming to EHP. About one-fifth of the workers began drinking heavily after their twenties; of these about half had been drinking heavily for more than ten years, and half for less than ten years. The majority of workers in this latter group had previously been drug users and had switched to alcohol, thus trading one dependency for another. For almost 70 percent of the study population, however, heavy drinking had begun in the teens or twenties and continued ever since.

Fifty-seven percent of EHP workers had experienced at least one instance of alcoholism treatment or counseling before referral to EHP. Ten percent had had alcoholism treatment other than Alcoholics Anonymous (AA), 26 percent had had such treatment in addition to AA, and 21 percent had been exposed to AA but had had no other form of treatment. This percentage of workers having had previous treatment for alcoholism compares with Smart's population (1974) of company-referred alcoholics, 51.5 percent of whom reported having received previous treatment.

With the exception of self-referrals, problem-drinking workers were referred to EHP under constructive confrontation and in that sense were nonvoluntary referrals.[2] Historically, the position of many alcoholism therapists has been to regard the voluntary seeking of treatment as an indicator of patient motivation and, hence, of treatment success (Sterne and Pittman 1965). Twenty-six patients (13 percent of the population) came to EHP entirely on their own volition—i.e., not under threat of job loss—and thus could be considered to be highly motivated. However, the responses of the remaining 87 percent to questions regarding their attitudes toward referral and treatment indicated that the majority of these patients were favorably disposed to treatment. Eighty percent felt that the referral was appropriate, and 76 percent felt that they had a drinking problem serious enough to warrant treatment. Only 15 percent thought that the referral was inappropriate, and 5 percent were uncertain. Similarly, just 18 percent saw

2. The strategy of constructive confrontation is described in Chapter 1.

no need for treatment, with 6 percent being uncertain. Taking both questions together, only 23 percent expressed negative or ambivalent feelings toward the referral, the need for treatment, or both. Thus, the attitudes of EHP workers at intake support the findings of other studies that nonvoluntary referral is not necessarily a barrier to a patient's acceptance of treatment (Smart 1974; Trice and Roman 1972; Gallant 1971; Schramm and DeFillippi 1975).

Age

Of the study population 12 percent were 20 to 29 years of age, 23 percent were 30 to 39, 41 percent were 40 to 49, and 24 percent were 50 to 64. The median age of referred workers was 43.2 (mean, 42.5; mode, 41). This median age is similar to that found in other treatment populations of employed alcoholics (Straus and Bacon 1951; Smart 1974), with the majority of workers (58 percent) falling within the 35 to 50 age group as expected (Trice 1959).

Race

The racial distribution of the study population was 61 percent black and 39 percent white, whereas in the Baltimore male labor force, the percentages are exactly the reverse. This racial composition distinguishes the EHP study population from all other reports of problem drinkers in their work roles, and consequently, in analyzing the EHP data, we gave special attention to determining whether there were any significant differences between blacks and whites in socioeconomic and work characteristics and in responses to treatment.

In a review of the literature on black drinking practices, Sterne and Pittman (1972) found that even in studies unbiased by who seeks or is accepted for treatment or by who is apprehended for alcohol-associated offenses, "Negro alcoholism and problem-drinking rates often range from one and a half to four times higher than white rates." The authors go on to qualify this statement, however, saying that "race differentials may reflect in part the gross nature of comparisons when Negroes are compared to 'whites' in general, rather than to other persons who occupy a similar position in the structure of American society."

That this latter statement may best characterize the meaning of racial differences in drinking and alcoholism is supported by multivariate analyses of treatment outcomes that find racial differences all but disappearing when social-class variables are taken into account (Kissen et al. 1968). Similarly, in the larger analysis on which this paper is based (Schramm et al. 1976), no significant

TABLE 10.2 RACIAL DISTRIBUTION BY OCCUPATION (PERCENTAGES)

Race	*Professionals/ Managers*	*Clerical/ Sales*	*Craftsmen*	*Operatives*	*Service Workers*	*Laborers*	*All Occupations*
EHP study population							
Black	27	41	46	72	70	78	61
White	73	59	54	28	30	22	39
Baltimore male work force							
Black	19	28	32	53	56	71	39
White	81	72	68	47	44	29	61

SOURCE: The racial distribution of the male work force in Baltimore is derived from the U.S. Bureau of the Census (1972).

TABLE 10.3 OCCUPATIONAL DISTRIBUTION BY RACE (PERCENTAGES)

	EHP Study Population			*Baltimore Male Work Force*		
Occupation	*Black*	*White*	*Total*	*Black*	*White*	*Total*
Professionals/ managers	3	14	7	9	26	19
Clerical/sales	9	20	13	11	19	16
Craftsmen	13	25	19	17	25	22
Operatives	30	19	26	31	18	23
Service workers	11	8	10	16	4	11
Laborers	33	15	26	15	8	10
Total	99	101	101	99	100	101

differences were found between black and white EHP workers of similar age and occupation in labor force behavior, job satisfaction, or response to treatment. Indeed, much of the explanation for the disproportionately high percentage of blacks in the EHP study population may lie in their concentration in low-status jobs, as will be shown below.

Occupation

Table 10.2 shows that among EHP referrals, as among the Baltimore work force as a whole, the proportion of blacks in each occupational grouping increases as occupational status decreases. However, as expected on the basis of previous studies of company-identified treatment populations, which consistently find an overrepresentation of low-skill-level workers (Trice 1965; Warkov et al. 1965), Table 10.3 shows that both blacks *and* whites in the study population occupied fewer higher-status positions and more lower-status positions than their counterparts in the Baltimore labor force.[3]

Since we do not have data on the occupational distributions of the referring companies' labor forces, nor a record of workers who were identified and referred elsewhere, we do not know the precise magnitude of the selective bias toward identification of lower-status workers to EHP. There is good reason to believe, however, that in the EHP population white-collar workers are even more underrepresented and unskilled blue-collar workers more overrepresented rela-

3. The categorization of occupations used in the EHP analysis was based on the U.S. Bureau of the Census occupational classification system (1970).

TABLE 10.4 PERCENTAGE DISTRIBUTION OF OCCUPATIONS OF REFERRED WORKERS BY TYPE OF EMPLOYER

EHP Study Population	*Industrial Employers (68% of referrals)*	*Government Service Employers* (32% of referrals)*
White-collar	1.5	56
Blue-collar		
Skilled	27.0	7
Semiskilled	34.0	2
Unskilled	37.5	35
	100.0	100

*Excludes the city sanitation department, which is known to have a predominantly low-skilled blue-collar work force.

tive to the population at risk than indicated in Table 10.3. As shown in Table 10.4, industrial employers referred almost no white-collar workers to EHP, and among the blue-collar subgroupings, the percentage of referrals increases with decreasing job status. In the referrals by government service agencies, employing primarily white-collar workers, low-status laborers and service workers would also appear to be considerably overrepresented.

Education, Religion, and Place of Birth

The median number of years of formal schooling completed by EHP referrals was ten. Fifty percent of the study population had completed fewer than 12 years of education, of whom slightly more than half had never attended high school. Of those who completed high school (35 percent of the population), 28 percent earned a high school equivalency diploma after having dropped out of school. Not surprisingly, occupational position reflected the level of education completed. Professional and clerical workers accounted for 92 percent of the workers (15 percent of the population) who had had one or more years of college.

Twenty-four percent of EHP referrals practiced no religion, 64 percent were Protestants, and 16 percent Catholics. Those who practiced no religion were found disproportionately among the 21 to 29 age group and among whites. Seventy-five percent of black EHP workers were Protestants.

With the exception of one individual, the study workers were all native-born citizens; and the great majority (95 percent) were long-term residents (eight or more years) of Maryland. Forty-nine percent were born in Maryland, 42 percent were born in the South, and 9 percent were born in other regions of the country.

Income

The United States Department of Labor's Bureau of Labor Statistics has estimated the current annual consumption budget for a family of three (husband and wife aged 35 to 54 with one child) to be $6,000 at the lower level, $8,920 at the intermediate, and $12,280 at the higher level.[4] In the month preceding intake, 36 percent of the study population reported a combined household income of between $500 to $833, and 54 percent reported an income of $834 or higher. Eleven percent had a combined income of less than $500, suggesting an annual income below $6,000. It is important to note, however, that not all respondents worked a full month in the period under question. In fact, of the 39 workers who reported earning less than $500 in the month before the interview, 29 had been on disciplinary suspension or sick leave at least part of the time. Of the remaining 10, 7 were service workers and 3 were laborers who earned a yearly salary of less than $6,000.

Social Stability

Investigators often use scales composed of marital, employment, and residential characteristics to describe the social stability of treatment populations (Straus and Bacon 1961; Gerard and Saenger 1966; Kurland 1968).

A history of marital disintegration has been found to be common among alcoholics, with the rates of separation, divorce, and widowerhood often exceeding considerably those of the population as a whole (Bailey 1961). At the time of intake, 49 percent of EHP referrals were married and living with their wives, 11 percent had never married, 4 percent were widowers, 10 percent were divorced, and 26 percent were separated from their wives. Of those who were widowed, divorced, or separated, almost half (48 percent) had been living away from their spouses for five or more years, and 37 percent from between one and five years. Despite evidence of past marital disintegration, multiple marriages did not characterize this population. Of the 184 referred workers who were or had been married, 84 percent had been married only once, and only 15 percent twice.

Eighty-eight percent of the study population were still working for the refer-

4. Total consumption in Baltimore City is equivalent to that of the United States as a whole. The city's consumption budgets exceed that of the United States by 3 percent (Branch 1975).

ring employer at the time of interview. As one condition for participating in the project, employers agreed not to terminate workers referred to EHP as long as they were in treatment and regularly attending the clinic. Nevertheless, 24 workers (12 percent of the population) were unemployed at the time of interview, for the most part having been referred by union officials with the expectation that they might be rehired if they could demonstrate improvement in treatment.

Of the 25 percent of the study population who were living alone, five out of six lived in conventional dwellings. Only eight persons lived in single rooms. Of those living in households, 68 percent lived with one to three other persons, and only 9 percent lived in households having seven or more members. For the study population as a whole, the mean number of household members was 3.8. Seventy-one percent of the population had been living at the same address for two or more years. One-fourth of EHP referrals were frequent movers, however, having made from 3 to 15 moves over the five years preceding intake.

In order to compare the social stability of EHP alcoholics with that of the comparison group of nonproblem drinkers from the same work forces, a seven-point scale of social stability was devised using the criteria listed in Table 10.5.

TABLE 10.5 SOCIAL STABILITY OF STUDY AND COMPARISON WORKERS

Study Population	*Comparison Group*	*Stability Criteria*	*Number of Points*
49%	76%	Married and living with spouse	2
46	82	One address in past five years	2
65	91	One job in past five years	2
26	17	Single, widowed, divorced, or separated and living in a family setting	1
29	17	Two addresses in past five years	1
19	4	Two jobs in past five years	1
25	7	Single, widowed, divorced, or separated and living alone	0
25	1	Three or more addresses in past five years	0
16	5	Three or more jobs in past five years, or unemployed at time of intake	0

As columns 1 and 2 in the table show, the comparison group presented a much higher degree of social stability on all three dimensions measured. With respect to overall stability, 36 percent of the study population scored 5 or 6, 39 percent scored 3 or 4, and 25 percent scored 2 or below. The corresponding figures for the comparison group were 85 percent, 12 percent, and 3 percent, respectively. While this may appear to be a trivial finding in the light of many previous studies on the social disruptions produced by alcohol misuse, much of the literature on working alcoholics tends to emphasize their high degree of social stability, often to the point of suggesting that alcoholic employees are even more stable than their non-problem-drinking counterparts. Such an emphasis seems more understandable when it is recalled that the discovery of working alcoholics was long delayed by the stereotypic image of alcoholics as primarily skid-row derelicts. Certainly EHP workers were far from conforming to such an image. Nevertheless, the above data would seem to indicate that alcohol abuse does have an impact on several spheres of life functioning.

WORK FORCE BEHAVIOR

It has been well-established that the productivity of alcoholic employees is inferior to that of other, non-problem-drinking workers with respect to quality of output and absenteeism (Trice and Roman 1972). Because absenteeism represents the most direct form of lost productivity, and also because it is easier to measure, it has received the most attention in the literature. Trice and Roman (1972) found that the absenteeism rates for alcoholic workers were from two to eight times those of other employees. Consistent with this range, data supplied by seven EHP employers revealed that the absenteeism of referred workers varied from 3.5 to 8.4 times that of the work forces as a whole.

In order to extend present knowledge of the work behavior of alcoholics, the intake questionnaire included many items on past and present work experiences. In this section we shall examine the work and task environments of study and comparison workers and compare the two groups with respect to age at labor market entry, job changes, occupational mobility, and job tenure.

Features of the Work and Task Environments

Investigators of industrial alcoholism programs have found that the risk of being identified as a problem drinker or alcoholic increases with the interdependence and visibility of a worker's tasks (Trice and Roman 1972; Warkov and Bacon

1963). This is a major explanation for the predominance of blue-collar, low-status workers in company treatment populations. Not surprisingly, then, when EHP and comparison workers were asked to describe their jobs in terms of five aspects of their work and task environments, the responses yielded a picture of workers performing highly defined tasks dependent upon supervision and interdependent with the work of others. More than 80 percent of both groups of respondents worked in departments of 20 or more workers and performed their jobs in cooperation with others. Over 90 percent worked a fixed time schedule, had no supervisory role, and experienced no ambiguity regarding what was required of them.

Work History

Thirteen percent more EHP than comparison workers held their first jobs before age 18, even though the median number of years of formal schooling was the same for both groups. The difference is explained by more EHP than comparison workers having held part-time jobs at an earlier age, suggesting less stable economic and social circumstances in the families of study workers while they were growing up. In fact, such concomitants of early labor-force entry as loss of a parent and financial hardship have led some investigators to argue that entering the work force at an early age may be a precursor of alcohol dependency (Perry et al. 1970).

Twenty percent of the study population and 39 percent of the comparison group had had only one full-time employer since entering the civilian labor force. Sixty-five percent of EHP and 91 percent of control workers had only one employer in the five years before interview. Thus, more comparison than study workers had spent the better part of their working careers with the employer they were working for at the time of interview, although the tendency to settle into one job perceived as providing a secure future and steady income was characteristic of both populations. Of those who had held previous jobs, 66 percent of study and 64 percent of comparison workers gave more money, job security, or better working conditions as the reason for leaving their previous employers. Only 6 percent of study and 7 percent of comparison workers mentioned work content as a reason for changing jobs.

A British survey of 300 recently employed alcoholics found the majority to have work histories characterized by no occupational advancement, and even by downward mobility (Edwards et al. 1967). For 59 percent of study workers the most recent change in employer involved no change in occupational status; 23 percent moved into a higher occupational status, and 18 percent moved into a lower one.[5] Although these figures suggest little occupational mobility, the experience of comparison workers did not differ significantly: 60 percent had no change, 28 percent moved upward, and 12 percent moved downward.

While the majority of workers in both groups had been working for many years for the same employer and, for the most part, at the same occupational level they held with previous employers, they had not necessarily worked at the same job. Forty-two percent of the study population had continued in the same job they had when first joining the company, but 30 percent reported having had three or more different jobs. Comparison workers, however, reported more job changes with their present employer, with the number of job changes increasing in direct proportion to years on the job for both groups.

The absence of upward occupational mobility among both groups of workers is consistent with sociological studies of intergenerational mobility which show that workers evince a strong tendency to hold occupations similar to those of their fathers. While there are shifts from one occupational group to another, especially in the lower strata, these are, on the whole, shifts to positions of similar status (Lipsit and Bendix 1959; Robinson 1969). At the time of interview, 49 percent of the study workers and 45 percent of the comparison group were working in occupations similar to those held by their fathers. Thirty-six percent of study and 38 percent of comparison workers held a higher position than their fathers, with the majority of these being skilled or semiskilled blue-collar workers whose fathers were laborers.

Thus, although EHP referrals had reported many years of heavy drinking and a majority had been treated for alcoholism before being referred to EHP, their work histories showed little evidence of a pattern of downward mobility when viewed against the experiences of their non-problem-drinking counterparts in the same work force.

Job Tenure

Previous investigators have found that frequent job turnover is not a characteristic of alcoholic employees (Trice 1962; Straus and Bacon 1951). Indeed, Warkov and Bacon (1965) found that workers whom supervisors identified as problem drinkers had longer job tenure than their non-problem-drinking counterparts in the same work force.

The median job tenure of EHP workers was ten years, with 53 percent having

5. This discussion of occupational mobility recognizes four occupational status levels: unskilled occupations (laborers and service workers), semiskilled and skilled occupations (craftsmen and operatives), clerical workers, and professionals/managers.

worked for the referring employer for ten years or longer. Although the job tenure of EHP workers was longer than that of male workers of similar age in the U.S. labor force (Hayghe 1974), the median job tenure of the comparison workers (20 years) was twice as long as that of study workers, with 76 percent having been on the same job for ten years or more. Moreover, 16 percent of EHP workers had been on the job for two years or less, compared with only 2 percent of comparison workers. The difference in job tenure between the study and comparison workers was pronounced, regardless of age, occupation, or race.

While the comparison group might appear to have atypical longevity, Siassi et al. (1973), using a probability sample of 937 auto workers to survey the drinking practices of United Automobile Workers (UAW) members in Baltimore, found the average number of years at the present job to be 13.5. Since the median age of these UAW members was 40, compared with 47 for the control group, a median tenure of 20 years for control workers seems credible. Moreover, information on the job tenure and age of the work forces of the eight participating employers who supplied such data indicates that relatively long job tenure is a characteristic of the population at risk; median job tenure ranged from 7.2 to 12.5 years, and the median age from 32 to 39.9. These company-reported figures are also instructive with respect to the job tenure reported by the study population. For only one of the eight employers did the job tenure of EHP workers exceed that of the work force from which they were referred; for the other seven companies, the tenure of EHP workers was somewhat shorter than for all employees, even though the latter tended to be somewhat younger than EHP workers.

In sum, even though these findings show no pattern of frequent job turnover among EHP referrals, neither do they suggest a population of alcoholic workers settling inflexibly into their jobs while non-problem-drinking peers move on to better opportunities elsewhere. Rather, the job tenure of study workers was actually shorter than would be expected on the basis of the length of tenure of workers of similar age and occupation in the same labor force.

JOB AND LIFE SATISFACTION

The purpose of this section of the paper is to determine whether alcoholic workers report greater job dissatisfaction than nonalcoholics in similar work environments. Although a number of investigators have hypothesized a link between job dissatisfaction and drug and alcohol abuse, the evidence is largely conjectural.[6]

6. For a discussion of the literature on etiological factors in work roles, see Chapter 1 in this book.

Consequently, study and comparison workers were asked a range of questions designed to measure their attitudes towards their jobs with respect to overall satisfaction as well as satisfaction with selected aspects of their work and task environments. Additionally, because a number of earlier studies have found some evidence of thwarted occupational and life-goal attainment among alcoholics, study and comparison workers' responses to questions pertinent to goal attainment are also compared in this section.

Job Satisfaction

Responses to two questions were used to construct a three-point index of overall job satisfaction so that we could compare EHP and comparison workers. These questions were, (1) How much of the time are you satisfied with your job? and, (2) If you were completely free to go into any type of job you wanted, what would be your choice?[7] As shown in Table 10.6, the percentage of respondents falling within each category was remarkably similar for both groups.

When these job satisfaction scores were examined in terms of age, occupation, and race, the findings were consistent with previous studies of job satisfaction. With respect to age, the consistently greater job dissatisfaction among younger workers and greater satisfaction among older workers found by other investigators (Gurin et al. 1960; U.S. Department of Labor 1974) was replicated in the present study. Dissatisfaction decreased and satisfaction increased with age for both the study and comparison groups. Indeed, workers aged 20 to 39 accounted for 65 percent of the job dissatisfaction among EHP referrals and 50 percent of the job dissatisfaction among the comparison group. By contrast, older workers (aged 50 to 64) accounted for only 10 percent of the dissatisfaction among EHP referrals and 8 percent of the dissatisfaction among comparison workers.

Researchers have found that the social-status ranking of an occupation predicts much of the variance in the distribution of job satisfaction scores. Professionals and managers show the greatest amount of job satisfaction, whereas low-status white-collar workers and unskilled blue-collar workers show the least (Robinson 1969). Consistent with the above expectations, in both the study population and the comparison group, professionals/managers were more often satisfied than the group as a whole; and in each age group, laborers and low-status white-collar workers were less satisfied than other workers. Although a greater percentage of

7. Many investigators of job satisfaction argue that simply asking respondents whether they are satisfied with their jobs produces artificially high estimates of worker content (Robinson 1969). Therefore, a second question, considered to be a more sensitive indicator of job satisfaction, was asked along with the more direct one.

TABLE 10.6 JOB SATISFACTION SCORES OF STUDY AND COMPARISON WORKERS

Study Population	*Comparison Group*	*Job Satisfaction Scores*		*Responses*
39%	37%	(1) satisfied	=	satisfied most or a good deal of the time, and if free to do so, would choose the same type of job again
34	39	(2) ambivalent	=	satisfied most or a good deal of the time, but would not choose the same type of job again
27	24	(3) dissatisfied	=	satisfied half the time or less, and would not choose the same type of job again

comparison than study operatives and craftsmen fell into the ambivalent category, the percentage of craftsmen/operatives who were dissatisfied was similar in both groups.

The distribution of job satisfaction scores by race was similar in both groups, and there were no significant racial differences in responses to questions on job satisfaction when age and occupation were held constant. This finding is consistent with those investigators who have argued that the greater job dissatisfaction among blacks than among whites found in several studies is a reflection of the lower-status jobs they hold (O'Toole 1973).

Given that only about one-fourth of the respondents in both groups expressed overall job dissatisfaction, it may be that the respondent's statement that he would choose another job if he were free to do so is a poor proxy for job dissatisfaction for these Baltimore workers. That this might be the case is suggested by the fact that when asked whether they would leave their present job if they could make more money elsewhere, 45 percent of the study population and 48 percent of the comparison group said they would not change jobs even for more money. Moreover, 30 percent of both study and comparison workers who said that they would not choose the same type of job if they were completely free to go into any type of work they wanted also indicated that they would not leave their present jobs, even for more money. Clearly, these workers did not perceive themselves to be free to change jobs, and the great majority mentioned security and/or seniority as the reason for not wanting to leave their employer.

A better understanding of the feelings of these workers toward their jobs comes from responses to a series of questions asked of the study population about features of the work situation that have been found to be associated with job dissatisfaction by other investigators (Vroom 1964; Sheppard and Herrick 1972). Table 10.7 shows that the percentage of workers who were rarely or never bothered by six features of the work environment ranged from 57 to 73 percent. (On the one such question asked of the comparison group—freedom to do work as one sees fit—the percentage distribution of responses was identical to that of the study population.) Even though 71 percent had little variety in their work, only 34 percent found their jobs to be boring at least some of the time. Of those who perceived little chance to get ahead even though opportunities to learn were good or great (40 percent of respondents), fewer than half were concerned about the lack of advancement potential. When these responses were examined in terms of demographic variables, the results were consistent with those reported earlier, namely, the greatest dissatisfaction was found among the youngest respondents and clerical workers.

Although a number of recent studies have reported higher levels of job dissatisfaction among the populations they studied (Sheppard and Herrick 1972), it is important to underline that the findings reported here are not at odds with those of other investigators. Overall, the responses of both populations would seem to indicate a fatalistic posture toward what they can realistically expect, rather than a positive feeling that the jobs they hold are among the best to be had. As Robinson (1969) notes, "To many of them [blue-collar workers], just having a job (which provides, besides more money, a certain feeling of membership in society as well as constructive use of time that otherwise would be wasted) makes them highly satisfied. This hardly means that they are ecstatically attached to

TABLE 10.7 PERCEPTIONS OF THE STUDY POPULATION REGARDING FEATURES OF THE WORK ENVIRONMENT

Work Environment Characteristics	*Great or Above Average*	*Moderate, Little, or None*	*Respondents Who Are Bothered at Least Some of the Time*
Opportunities to learn	69%	31%	34%
Opportunities to advance	34	66	38
Management's emphasis on quality of output (vs. quantity)	52	48	43
Freedom to do work as one sees fit	38	62	27
Variety (or lack of routine)	29	71	34
Amount of boredom experienced on the job	34	66	—

their jobs; rather their general mood has been well-described as one of 'fatalistic' contentment.'' That this may well be so for these Baltimore workers was shown in their responses to the question, ''Would you want your son or daughter to pursue this [your] line of work?'' Sixty-eight percent of the study population, and 73 percent of the comparison group responded in the negative. Moreover, even though more likely to find certain aspects of their jobs dissatisfying, clerical workers in both groups were much more willing to see their children pursue the same type of work they did; the seemingly contented blue-collar workers wanted better for their children.

The most important aspect of these findings, however, is the similarity between the treatment population of identified alcoholics and nonalcoholics in the same work force—i.e., the majority in both groups were not dissatisfied with their jobs and expected little intrinsic satisfaction from them. Despite the consistency in responses on job satisfaction between the two groups, there proved to be a clear difference between alcoholic and nonalcoholic workers in their assessments of their life achievements, as will be discussed below.

Expectations Versus Achievement

Previous studies on the relationship between alcoholism and occupational goal attainment have found that alcoholics often had job preferences at variance with the jobs that they actually held (Strayer 1957; Hochwald 1951; Hardy and Cull 1971). In order to determine whether a similar picture of thwarted occupational goal attainment would be found when alcoholics were compared with nonalcoholics in similar occupations, the study population and comparison group were asked how well their present job measured up to the kind they wanted when they had first taken it. Consistent with their responses to other questions on job satisfaction, 74 percent of the study population and 71 percent of the comparison group said it was like the job they wanted.

However, the first clear attitudinal differences emerged when two questions on overall life-goal achievement were put to the two groups: (1) Where are you now compared with what you hoped for when you finished school? and (2) Where are you now in relation to the things you wanted out of life compared with ten years ago? Forty-six percent of the alcoholic workers compared with 21 percent of the comparison group, or more than twice as many EHP workers, had experienced frustration in terms of one or both achievement areas. When respondents' perceptions of where they were at the time of interview compared with their hopes when they finished school were examined in terms of age, occupation, and race, from between 5 to 30 percent fewer study than comparison workers viewed themselves as ahead, and from between 7 to 23 percent more viewed themselves as behind. Similarly, with respect to respondents' perceptions of where they were in relation to ten years before, from 6 to 25 percent more EHP than comparison workers saw themselves as behind, and 15 to 35 percent fewer saw themselves as being ahead.

These findings do suggest a relationship between thwarted ambition and alcohol misuse, but the contribution of work-related goals to the overall life frustrations reported by EHP alcoholics remains obscure. Indeed, fewer than half of EHP study workers who said that they had not reached the goals they had had when they finished school reported dissatisfaction with their jobs. But why should alcoholic and nonalcoholic workers differ so greatly in overall goal attainment when the groups were so similar in their reports of job satisfaction? While this question cannot be answered on the basis of the data at hand, it may be hypothesized that although the majority of both groups of workers were occupying positions toward the lower end of the occupational status scale, comparison workers became more resigned to it by lowering their aspirations and finding compensatory satisfactions in other life pursuits. Or perhaps comparison workers had lower expectations from the beginning, never expecting great satisfaction from their life and/or work roles, and thus were less likely to experience frustrated goals. Conversely, alcoholics may have set higher life goals for themselves, and while not necessarily hating the lower-status jobs they occupied, were unable to compensate by finding satisfaction in other life areas.

Given the long history of heavy drinking reported by the study population, it might be argued that the abuse of alcohol itself was responsible for the failure of many study workers to achieve their goals. If this were the case, however, then the percentage of EHP workers who perceived themselves as being behind where they were ten years ago would probably have been higher. Only 18 percent of EHP workers said that they were behind relative to ten years ago, and 59 percent said that they were ahead. It would seem more plausible, therefore, that study workers had aspired to upward social mobility when younger, but were thwarted by larger societal barriers that act to perpetuate preexisting class and occupational positions. In fact, the tendency of many individuals in the lower and working classes to see themselves as fixed in life situations of relative disadvantage has been implicated as a major factor accounting for the poorer mental health found among lower status persons (Kornhauser 1965).

Even though the above argument is consistent with the hypothesis of McClelland et al. (1972) that heavy drinkers are persons having strong power needs, it is, of course, highly speculative. Respondents were not asked what their specific goals were, and it is equally possible that what EHP study workers hoped for when they left school was not upward social mobility at all, but success in more practical areas, such as greater material wealth or better interpersonal relationships. The data presented in this section definitely do not indicate a relationship between job dissatisfaction and alcoholism among industrial workers, however. What they do suggest is that investigations into factors promoting alcohol abuse in employed populations should examine job satisfaction within the context of larger life goals and achievements.

REFERENCES

Bailey, M. 1961. "Alcoholism and marriage: A review of research and professional literature." *Quarterly Journal of Studies on Alcohol* 22:81–97.

Branch, E. B. 1975. "Urban family budgets updated to autumn, 1974." *Monthly Labor Review* 98(6):42–48.

Cahalan, D., I. H. Cisin, and H. M. Crossley, 1969. *American Drinking Practices: A National Study of Drinking Behavior and Attitudes*. New Brunswick, N.J.: Rutgers Center of Alcohol Studies.

Edwards, G., M. K. Fisher, A. Hawker, and C. Hensman. 1967. "Clients of alcoholism information centres." *British Medical Journal* 4:346–49.

Gallant, O. 1971. "Evaluation of compulsory treatment of the alcoholic municipal court offender." In N. Mello and J. Mendelsch, eds., *Recent Advances in Studies on Alcoholism*, pp. 730–44. Washington, D.C.: U.S. Government Printing Office.

Gerard, D., and G. Saenger. 1966. *Outpatient Treatment of Alcoholism: A Study of Outcome ard Its Determinants*. Toronto: University of Toronto Press.

Gurin, G., J. Veroff, and S. Feld. 1960. *Americans View Their Mental Health*. New York: Basic Books.

Hardy, R. E., and J. G. Cull. 1971. "Vocational satisfaction among alcoholics." *Quarterly Journal of Studies on Alcohol* 32:180–82.

Hayghe, H. 1974. "Job tenure of workers." *Monthly Labor Review* 97 (January):53.

Hochwald, H. 1951. "The occupational performance of thirty alcoholic men." *Quarterly Journal of Studies on Alcohol* 12:612–20.

Kissen, B., S. Rosenblatt, and S. Machover. 1968. "Prognostic factors in alcoholism." *Psychiatric Research Reports of the American Psychiatric Association* 24:22–43.

Kornhauser, A. W. 1965. *Mental Health of the Industrial Worker: A Detroit Study*. New York: Wiley.

Kurland, A. 1968. "Maryland alcoholics: Follow-up study I." *Psychiatric Research Reports of the American Psychiatric Association* 24:71–82.

Lipsit, S. M., and R. Bendix. 1959. *Social Mobility in Insurance Society*. Berkeley: University of California Press.

McClelland, D. C., W. N. Davis, R. Kalin, and E. Wanner. 1972. *The Drinking Man*. New York: The Free Press.

O'Toole, J., chairman. 1973. *Work in America*. Report of a Special Task Force to the Secretary of Health, Education, and Welfare. Cambridge, Mass.: The MIT Press.

Perry, S. L., G. J. Goldin, B. A. Stotsky, and R. J. Margolin. 1970. *The Rehabilitation of the Alcohol Dependent*. Lexington, Mass.: D. C. Heath.

Robinson, J. P. 1969. "Occupational norms and differences in job satisfaction: A summary of survey research evidence." In J. P. Robinson, R. Athanasiou, and K. B. Head, eds., *Measures of Occupational Attitudes and Occupational Characteristics,* pp. 25–78. Ann Arbor, Mich.: Institute for Social Research, University of Michigan.

Schramm, C. J., and R. J. DeFillippi. 1975. "Characteristics of successful alcoholism treatment programs for American workers." *British Journal of Addiction to Alcohol and Other Drugs* 70:271–75.

Schramm, C. J., and W. Mandell, and J. Archer. 1976. *Workers Who Drink and Their Treatment in an Industrial Setting.* Final Report to the U.S. Department of Labor. Baltimore: The Johns Hopkins University, School of Hygiene and Public Health.

Sheppard, H. L., and N. Q. Herrick. 1972. *Where Have All the Robots Gone? Worker Dissatisfaction in the '70s.* New York: The Free Press.

Siassi, I., G. Crocetti, and H. R. Spiro. 1973. "Drinking patterns and alcoholism in a blue-collar population." *Quarterly Journal of Studies on Alcohol* 34:917–26.

Smart, R. 1974. "Employed alcoholics treated voluntarily and under constructive confrontation." *Quarterly Journal of Studies on Alcohol* 35:196–209.

Sterne, M., and D. Pittman. 1965. "The concept of motivation: A source of institutioral and professional blockage in the treatment of alcoholics." *Quarterly Journal of Studies on Alcohol* 26:41–57.

Straus, R., and S. D. Bacon. 1951. "Alcoholism and social stability: A study of occupational integration of 2,023 male clinic patients." *Quarterly Journal of Studies on Alcohol* 12:231–60.

Strayer, R. 1957. "A study of employment adjustment of 80 male alcoholics." *Quarterly Journal of Studies on Alcohol* 18:278–87.

Trice, H. M. 1959. *The Problem Drinker on the Job.* Bulletin 40. Ithaca: New York State School of Industrial and Labor Relations, Cornell University.

———. 1962. "The job behavior of problem drinkers." In D. J. Pittman and C. R. Snyder, eds., *Society, Culture and Drinking Patterns,* pp. 493–510. New York: Wiley.

———. 1965. "Alcoholic employees: A comparison of psychotic, neurotic, and 'normal' personnel." *Journal of Occupational Medicine* 7:94–99.

Trice, H. M., and P. M. Roman. 1972. *Spirits and Demons at Work: Alcohol and Other Drugs on the Job.* Ithaca: New York School of Industrial and Labor Relations, Cornell University.

U.S. Bureau of the Census. 1971. *1970 Census of Population: Alphabetical Index of Industries and Occupations.* Washington, D.C.: U.S. Government Printing Office.

———. 1972. *Census of Population and Housing: 1970 Census Tracts.* Final Report PHC(I)-19, Baltimore, Maryland, SMSA. Washington, D.C.: U.S. Government Printing Office.

U.S. Department of Labor. 1974. *Job Satisfaction: Is There a Trend?* Manpower Research Monograph no. 30. Washington, D.C.: U.S. Government Printing Office.

Vroom, V. H. 1964. *Work and Motivation.* New York: Wiley.

Warkov, S., S. Bacon, and A. C. Hawkins. 1965. "Social correlates of industrial problem drinking." *Quarterly Journal of Studies on Alcohol* 26:58–71.

ELEVEN / Job-Based Risks and Labor Turnover among Alcoholic Workers

PAUL T. SCHOLLAERT

In the past decade much of the attention given to problems which derive from alcohol abuse has centered upon the effects of this behavior in the productive sphere of human activities. It seems fairly clear that the heavy and sustained usage of alcoholic beverages is an important covariate of a number of work-place difficulties, including excessive absenteeism and impaired work performance. One facet of the relationship between chronic alcohol abuse and work which has received little systematic investigation is the degree to which certain jobs or occupational characteristics are conducive to alcoholism. While it is possible to identify certain occupations—such as bartending or the proverbial traveling sales force—in which the incumbents appear to have rather high levels of excessive drinking, it is quite difficult to determine whether it is actually the job which is causing this deviant behavior, or, alternatively, whether these are occupations which tend to attract persons with a proclivity for alcohol abuse.

Trice and Roman (1972, chap. 4) have developed a series of hypotheses which specify "job-based risk factors" for the development of patterns of alcohol and drug abuse among workers. Many of the suggested mechanisms which may promote deviant drinking are largely cognitive and attitudinal. For instance, they argue that ambiguous work-role definitions or prolonged isolation from one's family can create psychological tensions which may be resolved through excessive drinking. Several of the proposed risk factors, however, are functions of the structure of the work setting which are seen to be concomitants of alcoholism because they reduce the potential for sanctioning of an employee's drinking behavior by his supervisors or co-workers. Specifically, low structural visibility, irregularly supervised work, and flexible work schedules all interfere with the functioning of organizational sanctions against alcohol abuse. The worker who is on the road and away from other members of the work organization has the opportunity to hide his drinking patterns, as does the employee with leeway in setting his working hours or the individual whose output is rarely evaluated in any systematic fashion.

A major sanction for work-place deviance, including alcohol abuse, is termination. It is not unreasonable to assume that a worker who consistently exhibits poor work performance because of intoxication or a hangover might be fired for this behavior. But terminations should occur less frequently for alcohol abuse in jobs which protect the worker from sanctions, and thus, perhaps lead to chronic alcoholism. This line of thought also leads to a derivative hypothesis. *Among workers labeled as alcoholic, terminations should be inversely related to structural occupational characteristics which attenuate the sanctions against heavy drinking*. That is, within a population of working alcoholics, termination rates should be lower for those who are in jobs which are conducive to alcoholism because of the absence of consistent sanctions against excessive drinking. If the initial hypothesis is correct, this corollary should also hold because termination is an obvious job sanction. Termination is not, however, the only sanction which can be leveled at the deviant worker. Delayed promotion, outright demotion, wage cuts, seniority loss, or the denial of other benefits frequently associated with job tenure are possible organizational responses to excessive drinking by a worker. Thus, among alcoholic employees, one could expect to find that the incidence of any of these sanctions varies inversely with occupational characteristics which reduce sanctions against alcohol abuse.

Voluntary separation from an employment setting, which is the compliment of termination in the determination of total labor force turnover, is a function of many factors. One important dimension of this process is the vested interest which a worker has in a given job. As Parnes (1954) has argued, both formal and informal prerogatives increase with tenure on a job. Higher wages, promotions, and often better working conditions all accrue along with seniority. A worker who loses some of these perquisites because of sanctions against his alcohol abuse should, other factors equal, have a higher propensity toward job mobility than does the unsanctioned alcoholic. In other words, *among a group of identified alcohol abusers, voluntary separation should be inversely related to structural job characteristics which interfere with sanctions against heavy drinking.*

TERMINATION, LABOR TURNOVER, AND DRINKING BEHAVIOR

Alcoholism is not the only, and probably not even a very important, factor precipitating labor turnover in the U.S. work force. In fact, while the results are far from conclusive, it appears that turnover rates among identified alcoholics differ little from those of other workers, at least at the gross level (Trice 1962;

Straus and Bacon 1951). It is not clear whether termination accounts for a larger fraction of worker separations among deviant drinkers than among other workers, primarily because this is a fairly rare event in employment relations (Gallaway 1967). In any event, it is very likely that many other factors which influence termination and labor mobility in the total work force do so among alcoholic workers as well.

One of the most consistently noted concommitants of labor mobility is age (Palmer 1952; Batchelder 1965). As noted above, job tenure—of which age is a necessary condition—implies the acquisition of a number of economic and noneconomic work benefits which are usually not transferable to a new work setting. Married male workers are also less likely to change jobs (Gallaway 1967; Parnes 1954), since, presumably, they have greater social and economic responsibilities and, hence, should have a greater interest in work security. White-collar workers seem to have lower levels of mobility than do blue-collar workers (Bancroft and Garfinkle 1963). This is consistent with the presumption that persons with good positions—high wages and favorable working conditions—are less likely to shift jobs. Finally, union members are also less likely to experience job changes (Burton and Parker 1969). Unionized jobs tend to emphasize seniority as a method of benefit determination, and thus, long-tenured workers have much to lose in a job change. Moreover, unionized jobs are concentrated at the upper end of the blue-collar labor force, where higher wages may discourage turnover (Weiss 1966). Any examination of labor turnover within a population of alcoholics must consider these factors as well as job characteristics which prevent the application of sanctions against drinking.

Turnover and termination among alcoholic workers must also be considered in light of variations in drinking behavior. Clearly, it is oversimplistic to discuss the drinking behavior of alcohol abusers in monolithic terms. The methods, amounts, and consequences of alcohol misuse show considerable variation within any population of labeled alcoholics (Keller 1962). These differences in behavior may result in differences in the patterns of sanctioning applied at work. For example, some alcohol abusers drink on the job or come to work inebriated, while others drink only during nonworking hours. Some may be consistently drunk, while others are "binge" drinkers who become heavily intoxicated only at intervals. A long history of excessive drinking or a physical constitution which is particularly susceptible to the debilitating effects of alcohol may cause some workers to manifest unconcealable symptoms of alcoholism. And, of course, some individuals drink more than others, even within a population of identified problem drinkers.

DATA

The hypothesis that alcoholic workers in jobs having structural characteristics which reduce sanctions against excessive drinking should have lower rates of termination and job turnover than workers in other jobs can be investigated with data from the Baltimore Employee Health Program (EHP). Among the 161 presently employed male alcoholic workers with complete data files in this study, 58 men, or about 36 percent, had experienced turnover—i.e., had changed jobs at least once during the five years preceding their entry into the program. Of the 156 workers who had records indicating whether or not they had been terminated (fired or laid off) by the last employer, 21, or 13 percent, responded affirmatively.

Several variables collected in this program tap characteristics of jobs which, according to the arguments developed above, should be associated with attenuated drinking sanctions. Visibility is measured by two variables: the number of persons with whom the individual works in the routine performance of the job and the number of persons whose work depends upon competent work performance by the individual. The amount of supervision is gauged by a question which asks the frequency with which the respondent's work is checked (coded into high and low categories) and one which inquires about the amount of

TABLE 11.1 PERCENT TERMINATED OR CHANGING JOB IN THE PAST FIVE YEARS BY STRUCTURAL CHARACTERISTICS OF JOB

Variable	*Dichotomy*	*Terminated (%)*	*Changed Job (%)*	*Total No.*
Amount of job supervision	High	9.5	37.1	(132)
	Low	15.8	31.0	(58)
Schedule flexibility	Fixed	11.4	36.3	(182)
	Flexible	25.0	22.2	(9)
Job freedom	High	12.3	40.0	(163)
	Low	10.0	34.7	(20)
Size of work group	≤5	13.2	28.2	(110)
	>5	10.8	45.0	(80)
Number of persons dependent upon R's work	≤5	10.7	32.2	(87)
	>5	14.4	41.9	(93)

freedom the individual feels that he has in the performance of his work (also coded into high and low categories). Finally, schedule flexibility is determined by asking whether the worker is on a fixed time schedule or if he sets his own working hours. Also included in the analysis are a set of characteristics of the worker which should be indicative of his general propensity to change jobs. These include age, marital status (married and living with spouse/other), union membership, and occupation (white collar/blue collar).

Drinking behaviors are measured along several dimensions. Alcohol consumption is determined by asking a series of questions about the timing of drinking, and types and amounts of alcoholic substances ingested, all of which are converted into standard units of alcohol consumed per day. Each individual was also asked to report the number of years he had been a heavy drinker, the average number of times per month that he became intoxicated, and the general state of his health. Finally, each individual was asked whether or not he ever drank at work.

ANALYSIS

The hypotheses developed above were tested by discriminant analysis, a multivariate technique which determines the degree to which each of a set of intervally scaled independent variables differentiates between a categorically coded dependent variable. When the independent variables are dichotomous, as they are in this investigation, the method is analogous to multiple regression with a

TABLE 11.2 DISCRIMINANT FUNCTIONS OF JOB CHARACTERISTICS FOR JOB TERMINATIONS AND JOB CHANGES

	Standardized Coefficients	
Variables	*Job Terminations**	*Job Changes†*
Amount of job supervision	−.2447	.6262
Schedule flexibility	.2974	− .4975
Job freedom	.0539	− .2013
Size of work group	−.2332	1.4577
Number of persons dependent upon R's work	.2936	1.0156

*Eigen value = .029
†Eigen value = .036

dummy coded dependent variable. However, it is less sensitive to low levels of variance in the dependent variable, and, hence, is a preferable method in this instance. A full discussion of this technique can be found in Van de Geer (1971).

A simple bivariate tabulation of turnover and termination rates by sanction inhibiting job characteristics (Table 11.1) shows little support for the hypotheses.[1] Persons in jobs with high levels of supervision exhibit lower turnover rates than those whose work receives little direct scrutiny. Workers with flexible schedules are terminated more often but change jobs less frequently than those who work fixed hours. Since most persons fall into the latter category, these estimates may be somewhat unstable. Also, those who claim to have a high degree of job freedom have less work stability in both categories, although the large proportion of workers who claim to have much job freedom makes this indicator somewhat suspect. Those who perform their job with a small number of others (four or fewer) are more likely to have been fired, but they also show more overall job stability. Finally, the degree to which others in the organization are dependent upon the satisfactory performance of the respondent seems to be related to both turnover and termination.

When these structural characteristics of jobs are entered into a discriminant analysis of termination and turnover (Table 11.2), two patterns emerge. First, this set of variables does little to explain differences in termination and turnover. The eigen values, which tap the relative fit of the function derived from this set of variables, are .020 and .036 respectively. These are low and statistically insignificant. With respect to termination, all of the variables except job freedom seem to make similar contributions to the prediction of termination. Of these variables, however, only the number of persons dependent upon competent work performance by the respondent actually behaves in the direction specified by the hypothesis. The effects of these variables upon job changes are all consistent with the theoretical derivations, although again, the fit of the total function in explaining turnover is low. Supervision, schedule flexibility, the size of the work group, and the size of the worker's dependency network all have relatively substantial individual coefficients.

With the other control variables—those which measure propensity to change jobs and those which tap drinking behavior—the picture changes very little, although the overall explanation of terminations and turnover improves somewhat. In Table 11.3, the standardized function coefficients show that the drinking behavior variables are far and away the most important determinants of termination, and all of them, except the number of times during the month that an

1. The size of the sample varies slightly in various tabulations because of missing data.

TABLE 11.3 DISCRIMINANT FUNCTIONS OF ALL ANALYSIS VARIABLES FOR JOB TERMINATIONS AND JOB CHANGES

Variables	*Standardized Coefficients*	
	*Job Terminations**	*Job Changes†*
Age	−.1615	−.6015
White collar	−.1482	.2301
Marital status	.0069	−.1234
Union membership	.0856	−.4865
Health	.0117	.1423
Amount of alcohol consumed per day	.5056	.0903
R drinks on job	.376	.1003
Number of times drunk per month	−.4266	.2523
Number of years of heavy drinking	.4846	.0687
Amount of job supervision	−.2830	.2090
Schedule flexibility	.2296	−.1015
Job freedom	.0481	.0002
Size of work group	−.0969	.0950
Number of persons dependent upon R's work	−.2545	.1624

*Eigen value = .198
†Eigen value = .208

individual is drunk, fall in the anticipated direction. Also important, and in the hypothesized direction, is one of the job characteristics, the size of the worker's dependency network. The remaining functions are insignificant or operate in a fashion contrary to expectation. For example, the higher the level of job supervision among individuals in this group, the lower the termination rate.

Table 11.3 also shows the full model for job turnover. Age and union membership are clearly the most significant variables, substantively, in the inhibition of labor turnover, although several of the variables describing drinking behavior and job characteristics also seem to be central to the process. Job supervision, schedule flexibility, and the number of individuals who depend upon the respondent's work are all slightly related to turnover in the manner hypothesized above.

DISCUSSION

This analysis develops little support for the supposition that there are structural characteristics of jobs which protect alcoholic workers from sanctions against excessive drinking. Indeed, many of these protective mechanisms seem to be inversely related to termination, the most extreme form of job sanction. There was some minor support for the idea that these job characteristics inhibit labor turnover, but the noted relationships were small and insignificant, in both a substantive and statistical sense.

However, the theoretical contributions of Trice and Roman in this important area of industrial alcohol studies cannot be dismissed on the basis of the present findings for several reasons. First, there are clear difficulties in attempting to study a proposition concerning work history from a static perspective. The data utilized in this analysis were not gathered for a detailed investigation of labor turnover, and consequently, present job characteristics have been used to infer the attributes of past jobs. This is a tenuous technique which can be justified only in the absence of reasonable alternatives. Second, behavioral self-reporting is always fraught with validity problems, and this is likely to be compounded when the questions focus on deviant activities such as excessive drinking. Also, some of the responses to queries about working conditions are somewhat suspect. For example, an inordinately large fraction of the workers in this sample claimed to have considerable latitude in the performance of their work, a finding inconsistent with images of a highly regimented work force in modern industrial societies. Third, small sample sizes create difficulties for the analysis of relatively rare events like termination. The reliability of some of the estimates in this work might be enhanced with a larger study group. Finally, there may be other types of job sanctions, such as wage or benefit losses, not considered here which play a heavy role in attempts to control on-the-job behavior of alcoholics. It may be that employers are reluctant to use the ultimate sanction of termination with alcoholic employees and that the effects of drinking have inhibited the workers' mobility, so that the process hypothesized in this work comes into play infrequently.

A definitive test of the hypotheses developed above probably must await a longitudinal analysis which follows a set of workers through the life-cycle process of various occupational experiences in order to isolate the aspects of the work situation that are causally important in the development of alcoholism. Until then, judgments about the labor market and job forces which generate such behaviors should be taken with some reservation.

REFERENCES

Bancroft, G., and S. S. Garfinkle. 1963. "Job mobility in 1961." *Special Labor Force Report No. 35*. Washington, D.C.: U.S. Government Printing Office.

Batchelder, A. B. 1965. "Occupational and geographic mobility." *Industrial and Labor Relations Review* 18:570–83.

Burton, J. F., Jr., and J. E. Parker. 1969. "Interindustry variations in voluntary labor mobility." *Industrial and Labor Relations Review* 22:199–216.

Gallaway, L. E. 1967. *Interindustry Labor Mobility in the United States, 1957 to 1960*. Social Security Administration Research Report no. 18. Washington, D.C.: U.S. Government Printing Office.

Keller, M. "The definition of alcoholism and the estimation of its prevalence." In D. J. Pittman and C. R. Snyder, eds., *Society, Culture and Drinking Patterns*. New York: Wiley.

Palmer, G. L. 1952. *Labor Mobility in Six Cities*. New York: Social Science Research Council.

Straus, R., and S. D. Bacon. 1951. "Alcoholism and social stability: A study of occupational integration in 2,023 male clinic patients." *Quarterly Journal of Studies on Alcohol* 12:231–60.

Trice, H. M. 1962. "The job behavior of problem drinkers." In D. J. Pittman and C. R. Snyder, eds., *Society, Culture and Drinking Patterns*. New York: Wiley.

Trice, H. M., and P. M. Roman. 1972. *Spirits and Demons at Work: Alcohol and Other Drugs on the Job*. Ithaca: New York State School of Industrial and Labor Relations, Cornell University.

Van de Geer, J. P. 1971. *Introduction to Multivariate Analysis for the Social Sciences*. San Francisco: W. H. Freeman.

Weiss, L. W. 1966. "Concentration and labor earnings." *American Economic Review* 56:96–117.

CONTRIBUTORS

Janet Archer is on the research staff of The Johns Hopkins School of Hygiene and Public Health.

Ralph E. Berry, Jr., is professor of economics at the School of Public Health at Harvard University. He is the author of numerous publications on economic aspects of health care, including *The Economic Cost of Alcohol Abuse* (with James P. Boland).

Janice M. Beyer is on the faculty of the School of Management of the State University of New York at Buffalo.

James P. Boland is an economist with the firm of Policy Analysis, Inc., Cambridge, Massachusetts.

William R. Cunnick, Jr., is vice-president and deputy chief medical officer of the Metropolitan Life Insurance Company. Dr. Cunnick is associate professor of medicine at Columbia University and the author of studies on biochemical profiling of large populations.

Msgr. Joseph A. Dunne established the New York City Police Department's alcoholism program, which he now directs. He also is chaplain to the department and serves with the rank of inspector.

Otto Jones is the director of the Kennecott INSIGHT program and has served as a consultant to several large employers establishing treatment programs.

Edgar P. Marchesini is the manager of Employee Advisory Services at Metropolitan Life. Mr. Marchesini is a member of the American College of Life Underwriters and has served on the New York State Task Force on Alcohol Problems.

Leo Perlis is the director of the AFL-CIO's Department of Community Services in Washington. He has written several articles on alcoholism and workers.

Carl J. Schramm is assistant professor at the School of Hygiene and Public Health, The Johns Hopkins University. He has done extensive research on the economics of alcoholism and its treatment. From 1972 to 1976 he was director of research on the Johns Hopkins Employee Health Program project.

Paul T. Schollaert is assistant professor of sociology at Old Dominion University, Norfolk, Virginia. He is the author of several studies relating to the distribution of physicians.

Joseph Tramontana is director of special services at the Gulf Coast Mental Health Center, Gulfport, Mississippi.

Harrison E. Trice is professor of industrial relations at the New York State

School of Industrial and Labor Relations at Cornell University. He is the author of numerous books and articles on alcoholism in the work place, including *Spirits and Demons at Work* (with Paul Roman). Professor Trice conducts the Cornell alcoholism research project.

R. L. Williams is the director of alcohol services at the Gulf Coast Mental Health Center, Gulfport, Mississippi. He is the editor of *Occupational Alcoholism Programs* (with G. A. Moffat). Mr. Williams has served as a consultant to the National Institute of Alcoholism and Alcohol Abuse.

Index

Library of Congress Cataloging in Publication Data

Main entry under title:
Alcoholism and its treatment in industry.

1. Alcoholism and employment—Addresses, essays, lectures. I. Schramm, Carl J.
HF5549.5.A4A4 658.38′2 77–4783
ISBN 0–8018–1973–3

THE JOHNS HOPKINS UNIVERSITY PRESS
This book was composed in VIP Times Roman text and Optima display type by The Composing Room of Michigan from a design by Patrick Turner. It was printed on 55-lb. Sebago Cream paper and bound in Joanna Arrestox cloth by The Murray Printing Company.

HF5549.5.A4 .A4 CU-Main
c.1
Schramm, Carl J./Alcoholism and its treatment in i

3 9371 00028 5669

HF
5549.5
A4
A4

Alcoholism and its treatment in industry

DATE

JUN 4 '91			
MAY 31 '93			
FEB 28 '94			
DEC 04 '95			
NOV 25 '96			

45646

CONCORDIA COLLEGE LIBRARY
2811 N. E. HOLMAN ST.
PORTLAND, OREGON 97211

© THE BAKER & TAYLOR CO.